Confessions

of a

Caffeine

Addict

40 Anonymous True Stories

Edited by Marina Kushner

Foreward by Dr. Angela Browne-Miller

~ Praise for Confessions of a Caffeine Addict ~

"If you are an addict you need to ask yourself what is missing in your life that you attempt to fill with the addiction. So let these stories help you to focus on your lifestyle and behavior and help you to love yourself, your life, and your body." — Bernie Siegel, M.D., author of *365 Prescriptions for the Soul and Faith, Hope & Healing*

"Thank God for this book! The physical, emotional, and financial cost of caffeine on the public's health is staggering. This book will help you realize the dangers of caffeine overload and the benefits of reducing caffeine from your diet. Read this book and share it with the people you love. They'll thank you for it." — Dr. Sandy Bhasin, Chiropractor, Dr.Bhasin.com

"You don't have to be a caffeine addict to relate to *Confessions of a Caffeine Addict*. In fact, I don't know anyone without an addiction! Some of them, like caffeine, just happen to be more socially acceptable, but they all fall into the bucket of addictions nonetheless. What Kushner brings forth in her personal, poignant way is how addictions can be physiologically and psychologically gripping. I believe most people will relate to her heartfelt stories and extract a deeper, spiritual message that goes beyond even the bottomless cup of java." — Deanna Minich, Ph.D., CN, author of *Chakra Foods for Optimum Health and Quantum Supplements*

"Fantastic! Inspiring tales for anyone who ever had to face the very real symptoms of caffeine addiction. In this fast-paced world filled with sodas and espressos, *Confessions of a Caffeine Addict* is a must read." — Heidi Gunderson, author of *Migraine-Free Cooking*

"These stories will convince even hard-core caffeine addicts that they can end their struggles with caffeine. I know I'll be recommending this book to my clients who need a hit of inspiration!" — Alexandra Jamieson, CHHC, AADP, author of *Living Vegan for Dummies*

"Whether you are a recovering caffeine addict or just know one, you will laugh and cry with those who have experienced gripping the coffee cup a little too tightly. It's simply an invaluable resource." — Dr. Ben Johnson, co-author of *The Secret of Health: Breast Wisdom*

"Anyone who finds oneself medicating with caffeinated soda or that expensive cup of java in order to deal with stress needs to read this book." — Larrian Gillespie, author of *The Menopause Diet*

"This book is about real people, real lives, and real stories of caffeine addiction. It can be read in short bits and pieces, ideal for someone like me who doesn't get a great deal of spare time. Very well done!" — Denise Lamothe, PsyD, author of *The Taming of the Chew*

"It's not surprising that the most abused drug on the planet leaves a trail of addicts in its wake. These painful stories of abuse, addiction, and withdrawal should make you wake up and smell the coffee." — Susan M. Kleiner, Ph.D., RD, FACN, CNS, FISSN, author of *The Good Mood Diet*

"Caffeine is an addictive drug. These stories bear testament to the serious dangers of overconsumption and the major problems people face when they try to quit caffeine. If the thought of a week without caffeine gives you the jitters you need to read this book." — Patrick Holford, founder of the Institute for Optimum Nutrition

"Offers stories guaranteed to inspire readers to take a look at our stimulant-driven society and most importantly will encourage them to gain freedom from caffeine-based products in their diet. The benefits from applying can forge the path for creating vibrant health." — Sally Kravich, author of *Vibrant Living*

"Think you're not addicted to anything? It's very likely that caffeine, if you consume any, has hijacked your brain, your body, and your life. These alarming, true life stories will open your eyes to the possibility that caffeine is not as harmless as you may have thought. Can you go a day without any caffeine without suffering withdrawal symptoms? You owe it to yourself to find out and to take action to free yourself from caffeine before America's most popular legal drug will take over your health and your life." — Sheri Colberg, Ph.D., professor of exercise science, Old Dominion University, executive director, Lifelong Exercise Institute, www.lifelongexercise.com

"Reading about tragedy and recovery is the only way to combat all the confusion we hear about caffeine on the radio and from the media. These heart-wrenching stories give you new perspective on the drug. This book is not only an easy read but also it holds the interest of the reader. It's a book that you will read over and over again." — Archibald D. Hart, Ph.D., FPPR, author of *Sleep: It does a Family Good*

"As a lover and addict of coffee, I appreciate these stories. A must read for everyone living caffeine-driven lives. Wisdom is power!" — Darrin Zeer, author of *Office Yoga*

"No doubt we are a nation on overload, making caffeine an acceptable drug of choice to enhance our productivity. The least spoken about drug, yet most commonly used, caffeine can be as lethal as crack, cocaine, and heroin. A must read for all—whether you use caffeine to jump start your day or to simply accomplish 'just a few more tasks' to get ahead. Brilliant!" — Dr. Susan J. Mendelsohn, clinical psychologist, author of *It's Not About the Weight: Attacking Eating Disorders from the Inside Out*

"These stories about the potentially devastating effects of caffeine on a person's mind, body, and behavior show that caffeine abuse can ruin your life. Caffeine is a powerful stimulant and nerve toxin. It triggers significant biochemical changers, especially when your energy is low or depleted. Caffeine use should be restricted to the times you feel healthy and energized; otherwise it is bound to lead to an addiction. Take the stories in this book to heart; they are both horrifying and inspiring. We don't need scientific studies to know what is good for us and what isn't. These confessions are gems you want to remember when you feel tempted to overcome an energetic low by over-stimulating your body instead of properly taking care of it."—Andreas Moritz, author of *The Amazing Liver & Gallbladder Flush*

"As it relates to anger, caffeine is like throwing fuel on a fire. Caffeine tends to increase anxiety that often causes a lowered frustration tolerance. This lowered tolerance can often lead to angry behavior towards others. Caffeine should be avoided as much as possible." — Ari Novick, Ph.D., AJ Novick Group, Inc. Anger Management, ajnovickgroup.com

"I love it. It's vitally important information that needs to be shared. As they read, many people will see themselves and their lives messed up by caffeine and will be motivated to give it up." — Barbara Morris R.Ph., PutOldonHold.com

"As a practicing holistic licensed nutritionist, I have counseled many clients addicted to caffeine, the last of the 'legal' drugs. Not everyone who drinks coffee, sodas, teas, and energy drinks and uses drug store items is a caffeine addict. For some caffeine is a helpful nutritional addition. However, those sensitive to the negative effects of caffeine and are true caffeine addicts usually suffer from physical symptoms, intense coffee cravings, and have experienced a tough time withdrawing. Many will not connect the addiction with continuing long-lasting conditions such as headaches, fatigue, insomnia, lumpy breasts, mood swings, heart palpitations, urinary disturbances, and more. Many symptoms subside when caffeine products are discontinued. *Confessions of a Caffeine Addict* is an important read for those who think they may be addicted or those actively struggling with caffeine addiction." — Laura Zohman, MA, LDN, Cht Mind-Body-Therapies.com

"The average person hears the word "addict" and it conjures up images of street people with dirty clothes and cardboard boxes for their shelter. Well, America, this book gives you the true picture. In the 21st century the addict is the overworked Mom, the businessman and student trying to meet deadlines, and the truck driver forced to exceed his physical limitations. This book emphasizes how potentially dangerous caffeine can be. I encourage you to read and reflect on how caffeine works in your own life. I know this book will open your eyes about how nonchalantly this drug has crept into the American dream and for many people made it nightmare!" — Angie Lustrick, CN, CPT, author of *BODY By ANGIE: Is Your Body Bankrupt? Learn to Invest in Yourself*

"These stories serve to highlight one of the predominant themes I see as a holistic nutrition consultant—that of legal and even socially condoned drug addiction. As with any addictive process, this one often leads to dismal health; and worse—it is generally ignored because of its perceived benignity. Reliance on coffee and sodas for increased energy and mood elevation is something I see in my practice regularly. *Confessions of a Caffeine Addict* can help provide the wake-up call to those not yet convinced that healthful diet and lifestyle factors are better choices for sustained daily energy." — Jodi Friedlander, MS, NC, Board Certified in Holistic Nutrition-Bauman College of Holistic Nutrition and Culinary Arts

"Reading this book is an excellent way to raise consciousness, create dramatic relief, and promote considering the impact on others—all important processes of change to help move readers through the stages of change from pre-contemplation to contemplation and perhaps even preparation to become free of a destructive addiction." — Janice M. Prochaska, Ph.D., President and CEO of Pro-change Behavior Systems, Inc.

"These true stories will shock any frenzied caffeine addict into reality. Personal life experiences shed light on the dangers hiding in common beverages like soda and lattes." — Yvona Fast, author of *Employment for Individuals with Asperger Syndrome or Non-Verbal Learning Disability: Stories and Strategies*

"Combining caffeine and alcohol can trick the brain, making people think they're sober—or sober enough—when they're not. The stories in this book will make anyone think twice about consuming this dangerous duo." — Roy Eskapa, Ph.D., author of *The Cure for Alcoholism*

"Kushner points out the dangers of caffeine addiction, which is a widespread, underrecognized drug addiction in our society. From the omniprevalent morning coffee to the overuse of highly caffeinated 'energy drinks' by everyone, including school children, caffeine can wreck havoc on the nerves, as well as adreanal glands, which actually leads to decreased overall energy—quite the opposite of what the caffeine addicted are expected!"—Ellen Kamhi, Ph.D., RN, author of *Weight Loss: The Alternative Medicine Guide*

"This extraordinary collection of personal stories highlights a serious and growing problem in our culture, which has been almost completely overlooked: the overuse of caffeine-based stimulants to deal with our hectic modern lifestyles. Even when it's discussed, our preoccupation with caffeine is often shrugged off or trivialized while lives are being destroyed by addiction to coffee, colas, energy drinks, and pills, even among our children. Parents, teachers, truck drivers, workers, and just about everyone can benefit by reading these revealing testimonies about the addictive powers and serious health effects of our favorite drug—caffeine." — Randy Rolfe, JD, MA, author of *The Seven Secrets of Successful Parents*

"A vivid testimonial of caffeine addiction. A compelling guide to recovery and prevention." — Bruce Cortis, M.D., author of *The Spiritual Heart*

CONFESSIONS OF A CAFFEINE ADDICT

40 TRUE ANONYMOUS STORIES
Edited by Marina Kushner

Publisher's Comment: This book is not intended as a substitute for medical advice from physicians. The purpose of this book is to educate. It is sold with the understanding that the publisher and author shall neither be liable nor responsible for any injury caused or alleged to be caused by the information contained in this book. The reader should consult a qualified health care provider regarding his or her health. This book's contents should not be construed as medical advice. If you do not wish to be bound by the above, you may return this book to the publisher for a full refund.

Throughout this book, trademarked names are used. Rather than indicating every occurrence of a trademarked name as such, this book uses the names only in an editorial fashion and to the benefit of the trademark owner with no intention of infringement of the trademark. The author and publisher have made every effort to ensure the accuracy of the information herein. However, the information contained in this book is sold without warranty, either express or implied. Neither the authors and SCR Inc nor its dealers or distributors, will be held liable for any damages to be caused either directly or indirectly by the instructions contained in this book, or by the products described herein.

No part of this book may be reproduced or transmitted in any form or by any means, electronic or mechanical, including photocopying, recording, or by any information storage and retrieval system, without written permission from the publisher, except for the inclusion of brief quotations in a review.

ISBN 978-097475826-8

Cover design by Joe Potter Coffee Photo by Darren Hester

ATTENTION: SCHOOLS, NON-PROFITS, & CORPORATIONS
SCR, INC books are available at volume discounts with bulk purchases for educational, business, or sales promotional use.

For information, write to:
SCR, INC
93 S.Jackson St -46673
Seattle, WA 98104

Table of Contents

~ Acknowledgements ~

Our thanks to Amanda Curtis, Amu, Amy Doxey, Beth Anderle, Brad Justice, Cori Fay, Clare Mertz, TreSa Sanfilippo, Cristina Brooks, Dana, Elliott Riebman, Gina, Joanne Heen, Jennifer Bowen, Jeremy Johnson, Jennifer Knightstep, J.Todd Long, Sean Nolan, Jessica Kildow, Kat Koorey, Kate Marie Long, Marie Duffoo, Max Logan, Nalea J. Ko, Amber Welling, Rebecca Lloydjones, Sasha Gracanin, Scott Houston, Shannon Reinecke, Sarah Williams, Tracy Bagby, Thomas F. Shamma, Toby Tomulet, William Bales, Zachary S. Kaplan and other authors who preferred to remain anonymous for sharing their stories. We also thank Dorothy Sonntag and Margaret McIlnay for their contribution in editing and proofreading these stories.

Foreword

Caffeine: The Seemingly "Ok" Addiction

Perhaps the most overlooked of all addictions is addiction to caffeine. Coffee and other products containing caffeine are socially acceptable despite the all too common crossing of the boundary from casual to regular to addicted use (the progression which I have thoroughly detailed in my book *Rewiring Your Self to Break Addictions and Habits).* As caffeine overuse is so prevalent and even encouraged in our society, we rarely admit the extent of the health problems stemming from this addiction.

We tend to disregard, or want to deny, the fact that caffeine is the most commonly used psychoactive drug in the world. Besides beverages, numerous over-the-counter, non-prescription drugs for migraines, pain, allergies, and tiredness contain caffeine. The majority of adults on the planet consume caffeine every day at psychoactive dosage levels.

In my research, much of it noted in *Working Dazed: Why Drugs Pervade the Workplace and What Can Be Done About This,* I have found that parents, teachers, doctors, lawyers, and others not only defend the use of this legal stimulant, caffeine, they even invite its consumption. Furthermore, employers frequently encourage caffeine use, knowing that productivity can be at least briefly enhanced in employees willing to consume this drug. After all, what business interests and lobbies worldwide might balk, were we to point out how much money flows around this phenomenon—caffeine addiction? Most of the time, employers and employees don't recognize the damage caused by excessive caffeine consumption. When an employee finally crashes and burns, or feels the serious mental and physical decline, or reaches a point of "tolerance" where the caffeine no longer has the energizing effects, that employee is likely out on sick leave or fired for lowered productivity.

Many people do know the rugged dip, the tough withdrawal from a bout of heavy caffeine drinking. And many know the painful withdrawal symptoms that arise when attempting to stop ongoing consumption of caffeine altogether. Having worked with thousands of patients dealing with addictive substances and behavioral issues, I say that ongoing habitual caffeine overuse must be regarded as a real addiction and therefore taken seriously.

Caffeine acts in several ways to exert effects on the central nervous system. Caffeine crosses the blood-brain barrier with ease. In little time after it is consumed, the neurological effects of caffeine on the brain and nervous system begin to be apparent and thus are central to any discussion of caffeine as addictive. Caffeine's similarity in structure to adenosine, naturally present in the brain, allows the caffeine metabolite molecule to bind to adenosine receptors on the surface of brain cells. This results in caffeine's blocking of adenosine's access to brain cell receptors. Adenosine plays a central role in the transfer and regulation of energy throughout the body, however its useful effects can be blocked by caffeine—blocked in small occasional amounts for irregular consumers and in great and ongoing quantities for addicts.

The work of our natural adenosine is essential to our health and well-being. Adenosine is indeed a key neuro-modulator with powerful and essential effects on the brain, nervous system, and body. In essence, four types of adenosine receptors are present in

4

the human brain, all of which can be blocked by caffeine consumption. The functions of these four types of receptors include, but are not limited to: the general inhibitory function, which can slow metabolic activity when this slowing is needed, and the regulation of the heart's oxygen consumption and blood flow to itself and thus the body. Adenosine is central in the promoting and protecting of health within the body in the range of relaxation, suppression of agitation and over-arousal, adequate rest and sleep, and has valuable anti-inflammatory effects.

Every day it is becoming more clear that inflammation is a precursor to many chronic health conditions.

However, there are those who will insist there are powerful and positive effects of caffeine on the body. For example, caffeine's blockage of adenosine receptors most certainly can produce, for a time, marked changes in mood, moving a person toward the more stimulated range, reducing tiredness and stopping depression. Caffeine can produce, for a time, heightened mental activity, alertness, concentration, and increased energy. For those who are also addicted to other neuro-stimulating drugs such as amphetamine and methamphetamine, the effects of the primary drug of addiction can be immensely magnified for a period of time.

Amidst cultural, advertising, and performance-related pressures to use a seemingly "safe" stimulant such as caffeine, it is difficult to convince the public that addiction to this drug can have significant mental and physical health consequences. However, we are waking up to this reality and beginning to question the intake of this powerful and powerfully addictive neuro-stimulant. Caffeine addiction is real and is hurting us. I see this in my own work every day. At least half of all persons with emotional and behavioral problems that have come to me for help are addicted to caffeine. They are suffering from this "hidden" addiction and unaware that their problems are at least in part related to caffeine.

The contributors to this book, *Confessions of a Caffeine Addict*, with their honest and daring stories offer us a compelling insight into this highly overlooked and even denied condition—caffeine addiction. Read herein episodes of caffeine obsessions, mental disorders, physical ailments, painful withdrawals, cravings, hallucinations, near death experiences, and more. These stories are a major contribution to the emergence of realization that caffeine is addictive, even dangerously so. This book is a must read for everyone living caffeine-driven lives, whether we are direct consumers or just enablers, participants in a culture that encourages caffeine abuse.

Dr. Angela Browne-Miller (Dr. Angela)
author of *REWIRING YOUR SELF TO BREAK ADDICTIONS*
(Praeger/ABC-Clio)
www.AddictionStoppers.com

~ 1st Confession ~
Caffeine Blues

I was 20 years old when I married my childhood sweetheart, Paul. I woke up with the man of my dreams every morning and went to bed with him every night. I was in total bliss! Soon, we had our first daughter Amia, and a short 18 months later, our second, Brittney.

Life was great if I did not count the daily decline in energy that I began to notice. When I finished college, I began working full-time besides being a mom, wife, and housekeeper. I was pooped, in bed by ten p.m. and up by five a.m.

I had never been much of a coffee drinker, except for the occasional latte, but that gradually changed. A cup of coffee in the morning led to another cup in the afternoon, and then a cup in the evening, so I could stay up long enough to see my darling husband before I turned in.

Eventually I was up to five cups of coffee a day—one to wake up in the morning, one on the way to work, one at midday, one on the way home from work, and one in the late evening. We're not just talking average-sized cups of coffee; we're talking Ventis, the Big Ragu of coffee cups. Twenty-ounce cups of extra-bold whole bean Italian roast. It was my drug of choice during the day, except for an 18-ounce homemade Columbian blend late in the evening. Coffee had to be a gift from the gods.

Paul was the first who noticed my erratic behavior, but my three-year-old Amia was the first to say anything. It was her admonishment to "stop wunning!" Running? I hadn't been running at all, but Paul said maybe I should take her advice. I assured Paul that I was fine and that I hadn't had as much energy since high school. I was bouncing off the walls and loving it! Paul, on the other hand, was concerned about my newfound energy. I didn't understand, I thought Paul would be thrilled by my ability to get things done and be an active mom at the same time—not to mention a good lover. Wonder Woman had her Lasso of Truth; Thor had his hammer; and I had my coffee. Couldn't Paul see that caffeine made me a superhero?

All was well until I had my first "attack." The girls had spent the weekend with my parents, and Paul and I were able to steal some time with each other. It was mid-afternoon. Paul had gone to fetch a few things to take with us to Dockweiler Beach, and I had fallen asleep on the couch waiting for him. I had always been a light sleeper, and all Paul usually had to do was brush lightly against my face or bare arm and I'd wake up. This time, I jumped off the couch with a shriek, startling Paul so badly that he tripped over his own feet and landed on his wallet. His gentle touch had scared me out of my wits and made him think twice about touching me in my sleep again.

We didn't go on a picnic that day. I couldn't figure out why I had been so scared, or why I was crying. Paul sat in a heap against the fireplace. After a few moments, he managed to say, "Honey, are you okay?"

To which I angrily replied, "Does it look like I'm okay?" I didn't know what was wrong. I felt lethargic and numb, yet anxious and nervous.

"It's the coffee and sodas, Hon. You need to slow down. Can't you see they're driving you crazy?"

I wasn't listening. I was slow-dripping a cup of my best Kenyan brew.

"Hon, you're messing with your adrenaline and this caffeine is becoming toxic and addictive! Are you listening to me?"

I didn't want to hear it, "No, I'm not, Paul. Now leave me alone!" I said furiously. I meant it. I sat down and drank my coffee and wanted nothing more than for Paul to leave and not come back until after the sunset. He obliged, not returning until the next morning. Paul was always a mama's boy, and his mother had called to let me know that Paul was there and had slept in his old bedroom.

I had to prove myself, so Paul would abandon those silly notions of my addiction to coffee. I would take a few weeks off work to catch up on sleep and take care of the kids—without drinking a single cup of coffee. To prove my intent, I gave him the go-ahead to trash all the coffee and hide the coffeemaker that I'd bought myself for my birthday, as well as the slow-dripper that I'd acquired at a yard sale.

It wasn't until the second day that I began to experience really strong cravings for coffee. In the middle of the night my heart was beating so hard and fast that it shook me awake. I was frightened and rushed to the bathroom to splash cold water on my face. When I turned around, Paul was behind me. "What's the matter, honey? Are you feeling all right? You twitched and jumped in your sleep for most of the night, but I was scared to wake you up."

I don't know why, but I slapped him hard across his right cheek. He was shocked. I was shocked. I felt a strong urge for coffee. I made a beeline for the garage to get my coffeemaker and an emergency stash, which I kept in the trunk of my Volvo station wagon.

Paul didn't say anything as he sat across from me while I downed an 18-ounce cup of Folgers. He didn't even say anything when my hands shook so uncontrollably that I burned my thumb. I guess I deserved that burn.

This experiment didn't work. I really needed coffee and continued to drink it as usual, and Paul continued to pay regular visits to his mom and God only knows where else. It wasn't the coffee itself that pushed us apart, but the arguments that stemmed from his warning and my defensive retorts: his "just-watch-and-see" and my offensive "mama's boy" name-calling, which resulted in his big, defenseless eyes glazing over before he got up and left to mother's or elsewhere.

Paul never said anything anymore. Not about the coffee or anything else. I knew he wanted to warn me about my sour stomach, tell me that excessive passing of urine and weekly diarrhea weren't normal, or that I was cold all the time, even in Los Angeles in July. He never said anything when I gained weight (which was later attributed to an increase in stress hormones). Paul was a gentleman. I knew he worried about me because of my headaches, absent-mindedness (which was increasing all the time), palpitations, exhaustion, depression, anxiety, and mood swings—things that I'd never experienced before submitting to my master, caffeine. I wanted it, I needed it, and I was addicted to it.

I sat on the patio, sipping the dark roast and watching my kids play. I always played with them, but I was afraid that I was going to pass out and Paul wasn't home.

One day, I did pass out. I was at work early, trying to finish a project when I started to feel sick. My hands got cold and clammy, my stomach painfully cramped, and I folded like a napkin. I felt disoriented and lightheaded, and I could feel my heart thumping, thumping, thumping. I don't remember anything between reaching for my desk and waking up surrounded by EMT workers and the few employees who had come in by then. I refused to go to the hospital and stayed to finish my work. I decided not to tell Paul, but he found out and insisted that I make an appointment to see the doctor. I did the next day.

Dr. Werner ran some tests, did some blood work, and concluded that my symptoms were due to the over-consumption of caffeine; I was taking in well over 2,000 mg a day. On top of that, I was diagnosed with generalized anxiety disorder as a result of my caffeine intake. The doctor prescribed medication and advised me to give up coffee while on anti-anxiety meds, as the combination would cause my heart to race and abnormally stimulate my nervous system.

So, there I was, taking anti-anxiety meds twice a day, without caffeine. The problem was that the medication made me sleepy, and coffee had always been my cure for lethargy. When I threw caution to the wind and consumed both, my heart raced so fast that I knew it was all going to be over. All I could think about was my kids…and Paul. He had taken Amia and Britt to his sister's in Sacramento for a week to give me time to get myself together.

When my heart finally settled, I threw out the coffeemakers and tossed the coffee into the trash bin in the backyard. I cried and cried and wondered how I had arrived at this place.

When Paul served me with divorce papers, everyone else was shocked, but not me. Love dies from the wrong word, the wrong glance. Our family and friends knew we had been at odds over my caffeine habit, but it was just coffee! Who divorces over coffee?

Two-and-a-half years have passed since the divorce, and I'm off the anti-anxiety meds and have a can of soda every now and then.

When I think of it all, over a sensible cup of green tea, I remember that it all started with a cup of coffee.

~ 2nd Confession ~
Unforgettable Ride

For years I drove 18-wheelers coast to coast. Sometimes I would start in Norfolk, Virginia, sometimes in Memphis, Tennessee. No matter where, all I ever needed was caffeine to help me get from sea to shining sea. I was one of those guys they gave the load to when it was already late and had to be there yesterday. I liked the challenge. It was a game to me, played with 80,000-pound toys, a sport if you will, rolling way over the legal speed limit. The game was to get there on time, and I always played with the clock against me. There were many other pitfalls along the way, too, such as bad weather, scales I wanted to avoid, "bears" who would give out speeding tickets, or, worse, check your log book and put you out of service for driving too many hours.

It was remembering where to turn off to get around the scales. It was remembering which of your several log books you were using at any particular time. It was keeping manifestos and fuel loading slips in proper order. It was making sure you kept one ear cocked to the CB, so you could keep up with what was going on 20, 50, or 100 miles ahead and plan your trip from the Rand McNally in your lap, while you were eating a sandwich, all at 85+ mph.

I didn't drive just from coast to coast. I drove from coast to coast to coast—from the Atlantic to the Pacific and back in one week. The biggest problem I had, and all drivers had, was staying awake. Sure, you could doze at the wheel. After all, you were driving down a 25-foot-wide ribbon of concrete; any jockey could do that. So what did we use to keep conscious, if not totally awake? Most truckers use caffeine, mainly since federal trucking regulations require random mandatory drug testing, and that could take place at your home terminal, at any scale house, or on a whim as a call from your friendly dispatcher. But nothing forbids caffeine, even in amounts sufficient to wire an elephant. So that is what I used, each day, each week, every trip.

The trip started for me at the fuel island. I would fill my thermos with coffee straight from the pot, no cream or sweetener. Sugar would give me a quick rush, but would make me crash just as fast, and I sure didn't want that. Cream would dilute the effect of caffeine. Somewhere close to the fuel desk would be half a dozen brands of caffeine pills, and I would buy a pocketful of those. If I was lucky, the store would carry Jolt cola. Together with a few sandwiches, I was ready to roll, and three days later I would be on the opposite coast.

When I started driving 18-wheelers, I already knew that the cardinal sin was not being able to deliver on time. I wanted to do well. I came from a family of truckers. My daddy, my uncles, and my big brother were all truckers. Truck driving was not a job; it was a lifestyle. They each had their own truck, and more than anything I wanted one of my own. On those rare family get-togethers, it was all about where you had been, what you hauled, and how fast you got it there. That is the main goal of a truck driver. Do whatever it takes to deliver on time.

Nothing else mattered.

I learned early on that the legal way to remain awake and alert was to use caffeine, primarily coffee, and lots of it. If coffee was not available, then tea, soda, or pills would do the trick. Being wired is a familiar feeling for every caffeine addict: electric tingles, fast heart rate, and pounding blood pressure along with the dreaded red ear syndrome.

Whatever your reason is for getting wired, whether it be just for kicks or to stay awake delivering a load, if you don't keep yourself wired, the effects wear off. That is when the abuse begins because otherwise you will crash. I knew when I needed more since I did not want to crash. I got to the point that I knew how many cups of coffee it would take to get me through as many hours as I wanted to stay awake. I also knew that I could take pills for that extra kick. When Starbucks went nationwide, I could get shots of espresso along with my thermos of coffee.

Finally, I got to the point where all I wanted was espresso.

By that time I could not start my day without caffeine. Some people I knew would smoke a cigarette sitting on the side of their bed first thing every morning. Instead, I would walk inside the truck stop where I spent the night and have my first cup of coffee. That is how I started my day, everyday. I slowly reached the point where I no longer got a rush. I would wash my breakfast down with several more cups. Before I left the truck stop, I would fill my thermos. Sometimes I would drink two thermoses of coffee a day, plus tea for lunch and supper. Throw in the occasional soda and a handful of pills, and you get the idea of the monkey on my back.

The end came one winter morning in New Mexico. I was headed west and, as usual, running hard. I was flying low and fast with the sun coming up in my rearview mirrors, and the white snow showing off the many colors of the Painted Desert. They say a man can go to sleep with his eyes open, and I agree. My body quit responding to the caffeine and shut down. Fortunately, there was no one else close by at the time.

I watched through sleep-closed open eyes as the right front wheel of my long nose Peterbilt caught the soft earth on the side of the road and pulled me off I-40 and onto the desert floor. I couldn't have left the road at a better time. There was nothing to keep me on the road: no ditch, no fence, nothing to hit. I woke up doing nearly 100 mph across the desert in an 18-wheeler. Folks, it's a ride I'll never forget.

Growing up, roller coasters were my idea of the ultimate thrill, and as I crisscrossed the continent in my truck, I stopped at every major theme park and rode their roller coasters. There is nothing, and I do mean nothing, that can even start to come close to waking up in an 18-wheeler doing 100 mph across hard-packed dirt.

The great caffeine spirit had not deserted me yet. As if to compensate for worshiping it faithfully for so many years, the caffeine spirit kept my truck from turning over, slowed it down, and eventually stopped it a quarter mile off the highway. I waited there long enough for another driver to stop, pull over, and walk all the way to my truck to check on me. Finally, after pulling my quivering, shaking self together and assuring him I was okay, I drove back to the highway and down the road to the next truck stop where I went to sleep. For the first time ever, I was late for a delivery.

Knowing what caused the accident and that I had been phenomenally fortunate, I decided this lifestyle was no longer for me. I booked a slow trip back home, took my time, drove legally, and thought a lot. I knew that caffeine had to go and that the next time…well, there couldn't be a next time; the odds were too great against surviving it.

I returned home before the bad part began. I had no idea that caffeine withdrawal would be so difficult. I thought that withdrawal was only associated with heavy drugs. I was edgy with everyone. I stayed awake for long periods of time, unable to sleep, and then would finally pass out. At other times, I would suddenly fall asleep sitting in a chair. My body didn't know what was going on and was seeking equilibrium. My hands and my entire body shook, and my vision became blurry.

Gradually, the shakes went away, my vision cleared, and my stomach shrank back to a normal size. Acid reflux disappeared. And I swear that the hair on my head started to grow back.

Quitting cold turkey was not easy, but it was the only way I knew how to do it. I lived in the hills of Kentucky, where there were no clinics. Many of the little towns didn't have doctors. There were root doctors who brewed me herbal teas, which helped. So did long walks through the hills.

When I was ready, I went back to the only work I knew how to do—driving trucks. This time I did it differently. Rather than long hauls, I switched to heavy hauls. When you see a huge rig, escorted by police officers who are stopping traffic and shutting down roads for the load to come by—that's me. I don't have to get anywhere fast. I just have to get there safe. I no longer need caffeine to keep me awake.

Now I need steady hands to guide hundreds of thousands of pounds and to keep it upright around curves. Yeah, I may have a short cup of coffee sometimes on a cold morning or a glass of sweet tea on a hot summer day. That's all. I don't like the way it tastes anymore.

~ 3rd Confession ~
The Real Cost of Soda

When my dietitian used the word "addict" to describe me, I was shocked. Weren't addicts pathetic people who huddled in alleys, looking to score heroin or cocaine? But I was an addict—a caffeine addict.

Looking back, the ability to abuse was certainly in my DNA. My mother drank two pots of coffee every day. She was always on edge. The slightest noise made her jumping, gasping, and clutching her chest. She suffered from headaches and had a nasty temper. Come to think of it, everyone in our house was jumpy, suffered from headaches, and had a nasty temper.

While I was growing up, soda was taboo. It was in the house, but Mom kept an eagle eye on it. Milk, tea, and juices were okay, but soda was restricted. The reason? Soda was full of sugar, said my mother, and sugar rotted teeth.

I craved soda, however, and often would sneak a bottle into my room and drink glass after glass. Late at night, I would creep down to the garage and return the empty bottle to the case, making sure it was in the back row, so only the full ones would show. My obsession with soda eventually led to my addiction to caffeine.

When I turned 16 and began driving, I would go out with friends. It was the '70s and other kids were smoking, drinking, and experimenting with drugs, but we preferred soda and guzzled gallons of Coke and Pepsi. We loved the giggly, all-wound-up feeling we got. We could sit and talk and laugh all night long, smug in the knowledge that we were having as much fun as the juicers, potheads, and dopers; maybe more, since drinking soda wasn't dangerous.

In the mid-70s, there was a sugar shortage, so soda prices were very high. Sales were rare and so were coupons. One day a friend called screaming as if she had just won the lottery. She and her mom had discovered a sale on Coke. I ran to the store and bought six cases. I hid them in the trunk of my car, smuggling in one six-pack at a time, so my mother would not confiscate them. It was winter, and I kept the cans in my bedroom window between the screen and the glass. I drank a six-pack a night. Once a can had frozen and was all bent out of shape. I opened it and it exploded, spraying my face, hair, the wall, ceiling, bed, and desk. When I was wiping up the mess, I couldn't reach the spots on the ceiling and upper part of the wall, and they glowed slightly in the dark. My friends and I wondered what kind of chemicals in the soda made it glow. That didn't stop us from drinking it.

My whole family had always been night owls, and I was an insomniac. I also suffered from headaches. As I got older, I began getting migraines, and I was also gaining weight. I didn't attribute either problem to my soda addiction.

The first kidney stone attack happened when I was 21. It felt as if an ice pick was jabbing a hole in my side. I vomited from the pain. I called the doctor who said I had gas and not to worry. It was not gas, and I soon had my first ambulance ride. After a week in the hospital, the doctors told me to drink more water, introduced me to the healing powers of cranberry juice, and sent me home.

I spent the next 19 years being rushed to the emergency room many times for kidney stones. Women say that the pain is worse than childbirth; men just wince and turn white when talking about passing a stone. I was dutifully chugging my cranberry juice while continuing my romance with Coke.

In 1985, Coca-Cola introduced new Coke, changing the original recipe. I don't recall any rioting in the streets, but people were angry. Rum and Coke drinkers cried that new Coke ruined the taste of their iconic drink. People rushed around buying up old Coke before it went off the market. My friend Barb found a tiny grocery shop out in the middle of nowhere selling old Coke and bought their entire stock of 50 cases. She generously sold me half, so I was able to ride out the disaster. Eventually, Coca-Cola started offering both old and new Coke. Soon after, the new Coke was silently laid to rest.

My once-white teeth began taking on a brownish cast. Molars crumbled. My uncle told me that if someone placed a tooth in a glass of soda, the tooth would dissolve. I laughed, but I cut down on my cola consumption, switching instead to caffeinated, carbonated flavored waters. My weight kept creeping upward. I went on a health kick and cut out salt and soda and lost ten pounds. It didn't last. By now I knew that caffeine was causing my headaches, but I was caught in a conundrum. By giving up caffeine, I suffered terrible headaches and felt groggy. Staying on caffeine, I suffered headaches and was too wired to sleep.

The headaches got worse, and trips to the emergency room for kidney stones were more frequent. I spent years in misery and pain. I lost a lot of time due to kidney stone attacks and I lost a lot of money (ambulance rides are not cheap). One evening I went to the bathroom and the bowl was full of blood. The emergency room doctor showed me the X-ray of my kidney stone. It was huge; no wonder I was bleeding. The stone would never pass naturally. I would have to have surgery.

On the day of the surgery, the nurse said, "I bet you're a big soda drinker."

Surprised, I said, "Yes."

Then he dropped a bomb. "Didn't anybody ever tell you that the carbonation in soda can cause kidney stones?"

During many years of hospital visits and meetings with specialists, not even once was my diet discussed. Water and cranberry juice seemed to be the only cure for kidney stones.

I returned home with the firm decision to quit soda. It was harder than I thought. My hands trembled and even my voice broke. My head throbbed, I had dry mouth, and I was tired even after eight hours of sleep.

When I was weaning myself off caffeine, all those television ads of kids "doing the Dew" and magazine spreads of people enjoying "a Coke and a smile" were tough to see, knowing that I couldn't have any. I could buy a large pizza and get a two-liter bottle of soda free. Restaurants offered free soda refills. Who wants water with a burger and fries? Coke now came in cherry, vanilla, lemon, and black cherry vanilla. Didn't I owe it to myself to try these flavors?

It was hard to quit caffeine, but it was worth it. I haven't had a kidney stone in ten years. I haven't had a migraine either, and I rarely even get ordinary headaches anymore.

I was lucky I was able to quit; some of my friends and acquaintances were not. My best friend's mother who had been drinking a two-liter bottle of soda every day for years was diagnosed with diabetes.

Some of my friends have diabetes now; others struggle with their weight. A young man I worked with had a heart attack last year. He was 24. He drank two energy drinks a day, and prophetically said, "This stuff is going to blow out my heart one day." It did.

~ 4th Confession ~
Paying the Price

Many people overlook the damaging effects of caffeine addiction, but I do not. My propensity toward addiction started long before I started drinking coffee.

As a child, I subconsciously gravitated to anything that induced pleasure, which made me a perfect candidate to use and abuse stimulants. While other kids would sip on apple juice and milk, I had soda. Some days I would drink up to a six-pack a day, loving that wired feeling from the quick rush of sugar and caffeine. The better I felt, the more I drank. If I felt bad, I used soda to feel better. If I felt good, I wanted soda to feel even better.

Along with soda, my diet consisted mostly of sugary cereals and junk food. Chocolate also became habit-forming because my mom bought a lot of it. In combination with soda, my caffeine intake soared. Depressed, anxious, angry, rebellious, and paranoid, I tried to kill myself at age 13 by swallowing over-the-counter pain medicine. My mood swings became more severe and more frequent, and to counteract this, I consumed more caffeine, and eventually, drugs.

I started drinking coffee when I was in rehab I abused a lot of drugs, particularly heroin and cocaine. As a result I ended up in treatment centers 24 times. Every time I went into rehab and through withdrawal, coffee became more appealing. I also struggled with bulimia. When I was in treatment, I ate massive amounts of sugar products, especially chocolate, which I now know gave me a rush from its sugar and caffeine. After consuming so many stimulants, I would suffer from severe depression. I attempted suicide five different times. I also suffered from chronic fatigue, irritable bowel syndrome, and constipation. Caffeine would alleviate my constipation, but it was a temporary fix to an ongoing problem.

I finally quit drugs, but I became obsessed with appearance and food. I started bingeing and purging, over-exercising, and popping diet pills. I didn't realize that they contained caffeine, and I liked the rush they gave me, but I ended up withering down to 90 pounds. I didn't even consider the detrimental effects these diet pills were having on my system. I was more focused on my appearance than my health.

My life was centered on a quick fix. There are so many advertisements nowadays conveying the message: You have a problem? Take a pill. That's what I did. I had a problem—I would pop a laxative, or take an antibiotic, or swallow a diet pill, or drink some coffee. I didn't know that the very things that I was taking to help me with the depression, fatigue, and constipation were causing these disorders in the first place.

Due to my drug use, I became a homeless bum on the streets of Baltimore. I went in and out of treatment and suffered from chronic infections. Finally, I got on methadone and acquired a little apartment. My caffeine habit became completely unmanageable when I was on methadone. Caffeine helped with constipation; however, I started getting heartburn, nausea, cramping, and terrible headaches. My body became so dependent on caffeine that I couldn't have a bowel movement unless I drank two cups of coffee. The more I drank, the more my tolerance increased and the more I had to drink. Additionally, the methadone made me so sleepy that I had to drink a pot of coffee every day just to keep my eyes open.

Because of all the years of chemical, medicine, and food abuse, it had been about 15 years since I had a stable eight-hour sleep cycle. My doctor recently told me that this was partly due to adrenal burnout, a side effect of caffeine. The worse my sleeping was, the more coffee I needed. I was so addicted to coffee, and so tired from lack of sleep, that one day at work I started crawling across the floor to scour for change because I could not work unless I had coffee. I went around begging people for change just to get my fix. I would convince myself that tomorrow I would quit, but tomorrow never came.

When I came off methadone three years ago, I started drinking more coffee because my energy level had been severely depleted. I realize now that I was suffering from fibromyalgia, which caused severe fatigue, sluggish bowels, joint pain, and depression. My body was malfunctioning, and coffee just gave me a short-term Band-Aid fix.

I was ill all the time with bronchitis and other infections. I had hepatitis A, B, and C. The laxatives and bulimia had destroyed the lining of my gastrointestinal system. I continued to use caffeine, even though every time I drank coffee I would get a shooting pain in the back of my neck. I was so exhausted from my malfunctioning immune system, constipation, and adrenal burnout that I kept slamming down coffee. I needed coffee to function; however, because of drinking coffee, I wouldn't sleep, which took a toll on my immune system. I was so sick and tired that I started using energy drinks, which caused more anxiety and exacerbated my insomnia.

Finally, most of my bodily organs collapsed. I had a surgery that profoundly affected my already damaged gut, and I started going into anaphylactic shock from almost anything I ate. I could eat only organic vegetables because if I were exposed to pesticides, preservatives, or fumes, my throat would swell shut, I would lose sensation in my hands and feet, get a shooting pain in the back of my neck, and go into a suicidal depression.

I have fibromyalgia, non-diabetic neuropathy, Lyme disease, arthritis, liver disease, and inflammatory bowel disease. I am 28 years old, and because of addiction to drugs I have destroyed my body.

My addiction also led to physical, emotional, and sexual abuse. I realize now that I used to use caffeine as another substitute to help me escape from all my problems. The more coffee I drank, the more "up" I got, so I didn't have to think about everything I had experienced.

It has been five years since I've used street drugs, three years since I've been on methadone, three years since I've binged and purged, two years since I've smoked a cigarette, and eight months since I've consumed caffeine. I focus on the long-run solution and not a quick fix. I eat organic food and drink caffeine-free beverages. I see people sipping on coffee, which looks appealing, but I remember how I used to feel, and I don't want to pay that price anymore.

~ 5th Confession ~
I Have Chosen Life

For most of my life, I had low blood pressure. It didn't cause problems during my childhood, but in my teenage years I began to have trouble getting up in the morning. I started drinking coffee, and it seemed to help. I woke up, turned on the coffeemaker, got into the shower, and a few minutes later drank coffee with breakfast. By the time I was on my way to school, I was up and running.

Later, during college, I began to experience an afternoon slump. I figured that this problem could be fixed by drinking another cup of coffee. Again, it seemed to work.

I continued my studies in audio engineering and also took piano, guitar, and singing lessons. I formed a band; I played guitar and was the singer. The band was popular and we were booked for many school events. Our success led to opportunities outside the school, and we started playing all over the city.

Once we were booked for a Halloween party for a group of U.S. military personnel. Over two thousand people were expected to attend.

The morning before, I woke up with flu. That day was horrible. I ate nothing and only managed to drink some tea. I recovered a little by the next afternoon, but I was weak and dehydrated.

To make it through the night, I bought a box of Red Bull and drank three cans before the gig. The rest were positioned so that I could grab one when I needed it. That night I went through half the box of Red Bulls. The concert was a success and everyone was happy. I felt great until the effect of the drinks wore off.

I remember walking into my house, taking a shower, and going to bed. Two days later, I woke up in the hospital, with drips attached to my veins and monitors beeping, just like in the movies. Luckily, I was young and in good condition, so after a couple of days, I recovered.

I continued with my studies, music, band practices, and occasional dates. As I approached the end of my studies, I went to work part-time in a recording studio. The studio owner offered me to work as the in-house producer. I loved the challenge and did not mind the extended hours. What I could not do during regular work hours, I did at night.

I started to compensate for the lack of sleep by taking large doses of caffeine. Everyone in the studio was gulping almost as much coffee as I did, so I saw no harm in it. When I did not drink coffee, I drank soft drinks. I finished my studies and began working full-time in the studio.

Some of our projects became quite popular and money started pouring in. Many clients requested me as a producer. My schedule got busier. My social life was reduced to hanging out in the studio's lounge. Some of the girls I met at our gigs led to short-term romances, but nothing serious.

Years passed. The studio owner decided to retire and sell the business to me and my brother. We were ecstatic! The business became very popular. As time went on, we decided to move the studio to New York City.

By the time we moved, I was drinking about two liters of coffee each day. I worked 14 to 16 hours a day because the rent and power in New York City was more expensive. We needed to earn 25 thousand dollars a month just to break even. Business was tough, prices were plummeting, and we were in a frenzy. Some people did not pay and others did not pay on time. Money was tight, and we needed to work even more hours.

I was no longer a kid who could run on two cups of coffee each day.

The two liters of coffee I drank felt like water. After two weeks of 18-hour workdays, I felt like a train had run over me. I remembered how I drank Red Bulls when I was sick. I decided to use Red Bull for a week or two until the money from delinquent payers came in or I could hire an additional engineer.

It started with one Red Bull in the evening. The number of Red Bulls I drank increased. Just like a drug addict, I was convinced that I could stop at any time. I abolished water and drank only coffee and energy drinks. I gained 20 pounds and did not even notice.

There is no way you can drink so much caffeine and not be affected. I got about an hour of sleep a night. I added 10 more pounds to the 20 I had already gained. I lost most of my hair and developed an ulcer. I was unable to recognize the reasons for my problems. I was only thinking about the next bill, the next client, and the next check.

It did not stop there. I developed narcolepsy, falling asleep for a few minutes at inappropriate moments. I finally decided to seek help, still unaware that most of my problems were because of excessive consumption of caffeine.

I went to the doctor. I had not seen the sun in about a year and was very pale. He checked my blood pressure and it was through the roof. He connected a heart monitor and discovered an elevated heart rate. Five minutes later, I was in an ambulance.

I was happy to see the world, even through an ambulance window. I had not been out much lately and was making jokes and pointing out buildings I had never seen before. The doctor thought I was hallucinating. When I had one of my narcoleptic attacks right there in the ambulance, he thought I had a heart attack until I woke a minute later, continuing with the sentence where I left off.

I had to detox like a drug user. I had the shakes, temperature drops and rises, and blood pressure fluctuations. It was terrible. I was unable to sleep. The doctors did not give me anything to help; they were afraid that it might kill me. They had never witnessed such a high amount of caffeine in anyone's bloodstream. Four days later I passed out. I was asleep for three days. I continued sleeping for days, but with "wake times" that were gradually increasing. I was on an intravenous drip and even spent one day in the shock room. I felt drowsy, depressed, and useless.

A few doctors, along with a shrink, approached me one day and explained that if I continued my lifestyle, I would not survive. The shrink stayed, and we had a long talk. I saw him daily, and he instructed me on how to deal with the consequences of my abuse. I was not only a caffeine addict; I was a workaholic. I needed an extensive recovery time. There was no alternative treatment.

I went home to my parents. The more time passed, the less inclined I was to return to New York City. I loved my newfound freedom. I loved the spare time, the sleep, and the "take it easy" routine. I started writing as a freelancer. The money is not great, but I can work from home and do not have to rush or stress out. I refuse jobs with a "yesterday" deadline.

I got married and had a son, now three years old. If I had decided to remain in that vicious cycle in New York, none of this would have happened. I lead a peaceful life and watch what I eat because of my ulcer. I'm taking my medication and avoiding stress. Some of my hair has even grown back. I do not inquire about the business in New York. My brother is still angry with me for abandoning the ship, but I have chosen life.

~ 6th Confession ~
Caffeine Gene

They say addicts are born. There is a gene lurking in our DNA that gets triggered…and bingo! Your life changes forever. They also say addiction runs in families. My parents were alcoholics and heavy smokers. By age seven I could make the perfect martini. I could spell Pinot Noir before most of my friends could spell their own names. Of course, even with my bar tending skills, my parents never let me have any of my perfectly mixed potions, so I didn't become an alcoholic.

They did, however, unwittingly manage to get me addicted to caffeine.

I grew up poor, not trailer park and welfare poor, but there were circumstances beyond our control that ate up all our income immediately. When I was three, my mother gave birth to a baby boy who contracted spinal meningitis and then, within a few months, polio. My mother, until then, had owned a string of yarn shops in Boston, and my father was a bookkeeper. After my brother was born, my mother was unable to work, and every penny my father brought home was used for my brother's therapy and medication and my parents' liquor.

I remember suddenly learning that I could no longer have milk or juice. These beverages were now reserved for cocktails. Money was tight and the family needed to cut back on non-necessities. Apparently, my parents didn't think it was necessary for a toddler to have juice and milk. They had no problem in giving me coffee, however. That's when it started. I came to love weekend mornings. I would get up early to watch cartoons and wait for my father to emerge from the bedroom to give me breakfast. He explained that Mother needed to sleep late because she had "too much" the night before.

As my parents' addiction grew, my own addiction was beginning.

My parents found it acceptable to give me coffee and tea. Those drinks were cheaper than milk and juice. On cold winter mornings I looked forward to having coffee with my dad. He even showed me how to make it by myself. When my father went to work, my mother stayed in bed, and I was left to tend to my little brother. I would make coffee just like Dad had taught me, and I would put some in my brother's bottle, too. Even my mother took advantage of my coffee-brewing skills. When she woke, she no longer demanded only vodka and juice. She wanted coffee to go with it. I would sometimes sit on the bed with her as we shared our coffee.

Soon it was time for me to start kindergarten. My father explained, "You know how Mother doesn't like getting up in the morning. You'll need to feed and dress yourself and get to school on time." I did.

My first day of school was a learning experience. I vividly remember snack time. Ms. Smith placed one cookie and a carton of milk in front of each of us. As each child tore open his carton, I sat there hesitating. Ms. Smith asked if I felt all right. I assured her I was fine, but I asked if I might have coffee because I wasn't allowed to drink milk. To this day, I remember the expression on her face as she rushed me to the principal's office.

As I sat in front of Mrs. Fine, the school principal, I was asked to confirm my request for coffee. I said, "Yes, please." I even offered to show her how to make it. Mrs. Fine had the same look on her face as Ms. Smith. There ensued a short telephone conversation with my mother and I was led back to the schoolroom to enjoy my milk and cookie. My mornings at home, however, did not change. I either made my coffee or went without it. Coffee was nothing more than a beverage of choice.

During my junior year, a Dunkin' Donuts was built across from the high school. At lunch my friends and I became regulars there. I was beginning to understand the benefits of coffee. Until then, I drank it because I enjoyed the taste, or so I believed. I never felt that I needed it; although gradually I did realize that I couldn't function in the morning until my coffee kicked in. Coffee helped me wake up, function, and think. Studying was so much easier with a pot of coffee next to me. For Christmas in my junior year, my parents gave me an electric percolator to keep in my bedroom.

In the spring of my first year in college, my mother died. She died fairly young at 47. She knew she would. The alcohol and the cigarettes finally got her. She would tell me, "My only pleasures are smoking and drinking." No one wanted to take those pleasures away. Soon afterward, I began to experience severe, devastating, gut-wrenching stomach pains. I would spend days in bed. The doctor thought I was grieving over my mother. The nurse thought it might be menstrual cramps. I still had my coffee no matter how sick I became.

My father had his own problems to deal with. After he lost my mother, he plunged himself deeper into the comfort of Jack Daniels and became irretrievably lost in his own misery. I spent my time trying to comfort him, ignoring my own illness.

One day we had a career fair at school. I was feeling fine, but as I approached one of the tables, I was suddenly struck with horrendous pain, causing me to double over and drop my books. My friend Julie tried to grab my arm. I vomited blood all over her, the floor, my books, and me. The last thought I had before passing out was, oh no, these are my new shoes.

I woke up in the emergency room. "It's so noisy," I remember telling a nurse hovering near my head.

Without explaining my condition or assuring me all would be fine, she blurted out, "Honey, we need to find your father so he can consent to surgery, or you're going to die."

I pictured my father sitting at his usual spot at the kitchen table with a bottle of Jack Daniels. Before slipping back into oblivion, I whispered, mostly to myself, "Well, I guess I'm gonna die."

The next time I woke up, someone was softly slapping my cheek saying, "You made it. The operation is over." I quickly determined my condition: I hurt, I felt nauseous, and my head was pounding. I fell back to sleep. The following day I learned that no one could locate my father in time, and surgery was performed without parental consent before I bled to death. I'd had a stomach ulcer that perforated.

Assuming I had some issues at home to deal with, they sent a social worker to visit me. She introduced herself as Ms. Blaire and asked if there was anything she could get me. I wanted coffee. I wanted my comfort food. My mother never cooked much, so I never learned to equate food with feeling better. I did, however, learn that a warm cup of coffee always offered whatever solace I was craving. There was something cozy and comforting in just holding the cup and letting the steaming aroma clear my senses. I asked Ms. Blaire, "Can you find me some coffee? They won't let me have any." I don't know how she pulled it off, but she brought me a cup of coffee with cream and sugar, just as I asked. As she reached over to hand it to me, she noticed my hands were shaking. She said nothing as she watched me drain every drop. After we chatted about school and home, she commented that my hands had stopped shaking. She looked a bit concerned and asked me how long I had been drinking coffee. I said, "All my life."

She said, "I think you are addicted to caffeine and that's probably what caused your stomach to rupture."

"Addicted?" I was offended. I didn't use drugs. I didn't even drink alcohol. How can anyone get addicted to coffee? It's just coffee!

After another week, I was sent home with a strict diet that prohibited caffeine. I knew I was sick, but there was a limit to the number of sacrifices I was willing to make. It was bad enough that I had to restrict myself to bland, soft foods for a few months.

When our common sense fails us, however, Mother Nature usually steps in. Even a few sips of coffee made me ill. I realized I shouldn't drink coffee, but without it I had headaches, shaking, cold sweats, and bouts of nausea. I needed at least my morning fix. Before I had a cup of coffee, I wasn't even human: I couldn't think. I could barely move. A friend of mine told me that a NoDoz tablet has the same amount of caffeine as a cup of coffee. When it became unbearable, I would just pop a pill, reminding myself that I was not an addict. No matter where I went, I always had a bottle of NoDoz. I had lived like this for years.

Two marriages, two children, and several jobs later, I managed to find the perfect job that combined writing and editing, and I was thrilled. A convenient supply of coffee was an added perk. I was working in a building with its own Starbucks on the first floor. Everyone in the office took multiple coffee breaks every day, and we even employed a "coffee boy" to make hourly runs to Starbucks. I was thrilled to be working with people just like me. To make it even more convenient, our Starbucks charges would be deducted from our paychecks so the "coffee boy" didn't have to carry cash.

Too much coffee still hurt, so I had learned to control my intake because of pain, but not to control the actual addiction—a term that I still refused to use to describe my love of coffee. I would order frappe, frothy stuff topped with whipped cream. My stomach tolerated these drinks quite well, but my skirts got too tight. No matter how happy my tummy might have been, I had to find other alternatives. One day I ran downstairs by myself to ask what I could have that was light on the coffee and super light on the fat and calories. I learned about skinny vanilla lattes with sugar-free syrup. Bring'em on! These babies were 75 percent milk. I could have my coffee and make up for the lost calcium from my childhood.

On payday that month, I tried to pay my cell phone bill online as I always did. However, I got a message saying that we cannot complete this transaction. I opened my pay envelope and was shocked to see what my Starbucks withdrawals had been for the month. My bill was close to $500. It never occurred to me to start financially tracking my Grande latte consumption. I couldn't pay my cell phone bill, my car insurance, and my daughter's tuition. I would need to confess to my husband and ask for money.

During dinner, I tried to put a light-hearted spin on my little shortcoming. Not at all amused, my husband grabbed my arm and roughly shook me. He said he would not allow me to spend money on my addiction. There was that word "addiction" again. "For Pete's sake," I told him, "I'm not doing drugs, and I'm not spending my paycheck on liquor like my parents did." "It's coffee!" I screamed.

Our 16-year-old daughter walked in. "Oh chill, Dad," she said. "Rhonda's mom got caught doing meth. Mom's addicted to what…lattes? Jeeze!"

My husband was in computer sales. His commissions had dwindled dramatically over the previous months, thanks to the "dot com" bubble bursting. He was forced to withdraw funds from his 401(k) to pay the bills. He made me quit my job because even though I hadn't realized it, I had indeed had a major relapse and couldn't be trusted anywhere near a coffee supplier. I began working from home. He installed nanny cams all over the house to make sure that I was not drinking coffee. He even took my car keys away. One day when I decided that I needed some fresh air and tried to go for a walk around the block, his friend, a police officer, pulled up to ask where I was going.

While I was under "house arrest," my daughter tried to sneak me an espresso. As she placed it on my desk, my husband's voice boomed through the speaker, "Step away from the coffee." She laughed. I cried.

My husband tried to trust me again, but it was never the same. He said he could fight another man, but he didn't know how to contend with lattes and mocha frappuccinos. He didn't know how someone could spend an entire paycheck on an addiction and not pay the bills. He couldn't understand. We divorced.

I still keep saying "it's just coffee." However, I'm all too aware that the side effects are worse than occasional stomach pains and indigestion. A simple cup of coffee at the age of three-and-a-half had spiraled into a life long addiction that caused financial problems, loss of a job, and a divorce. Denial is no longer an issue. I am an addict. When I place my order with the barista who asks me, "Would you like an extra shot in that?" I need to close my eyes, gain composure, count to ten, and calmly reply, "No, thank you."

Last Christmas my daughter asked for a Starbucks gift card. I wish I could find that little gene in her head and turn it off before it gets out of control.

~ 7th Confession ~
Too High—Come Down

My caffeine addiction began during my sophomore year of college. I had a full load of classes and was pledging a service sorority. The pledging activities kept me up late, and I found myself sleeping in class the following day. I decided to start drinking coffee—just one cup. I would forfeit breakfast to get extra sleep. Why get up early just to eat breakfast when there was a perfectly good vending machine that dispensed the sustaining jolt of java?

The jolt of java strategy worked for an entire semester. I lost weight and gained concentration. I thought with one more cup of coffee mid-morning, I could sustain the effects. Then I added a 12-ounce can of Diet Coke at lunchtime.

There were no immediate problems. I only felt a heightened sense of alertness and energy. It wasn't until I had finished pledging the sorority that I began to notice problems. I no longer had the need to stay up late, but I could not fall asleep. I would stay up drinking coffee and study. Then I would fall asleep, but I wouldn't stay asleep for long. I would get up frequently to use the bathroom. During a day I also frequently ran to the bathroom. I didn't know caffeine had a diuretic effect. I was beginning to suffer from diarrhea.

After weeks of sleep deprivation and dehydration, I noticed changes in my appearance. The dark circles under my eyes deepened and my lips became chapped and peeling. By this time,

I had gone from two cups of coffee to five cups each morning and increased my consumption of soda. Whenever I felt a drop in energy, I had a cup of coffee or a can of soda. I constantly had a slight jittery feeling, but I interpreted it as energy.

I was always anxious and found it difficult to concentrate when I read or spoke to someone. I was not in a peaceful state of mind. I was irritable and impatient and preferred to be alone, partially to ensure that I would have access to my next cup of coffee. Caffeine engulfed me to the point that nothing else mattered—none of my mental and physical symptoms. I had some idea of what was causing my disorders, but I did not care. My day-to-day routine, doing what I needed to keep going, was all that I felt really mattered.

It took a while to realize that I didn't want to be reliant on caffeine.

Once I admitted to myself that I had a problem, I wanted to learn more about caffeine and how it affects the body, so I searched the Internet.

I learned that caffeine is the common name for a chemical known as the 1, 3, 7-trimethylxanthine, which is found naturally in over 60 different plants and also can be produced synthetically. In its pure state caffeine is a slightly bitter white powder. Just like cocaine and heroin, I thought.

I learned that a moderate daily intake of caffeine is considered to be between 130-300 mg. The average amount in an 8-ounce cup of coffee is about 135 mg. I was consuming well over eight cups of coffee, plus untold amounts of Diet Coke each day, which contains 46.5 mg of caffeine per can, and sometimes I took Vivarin, popular on college campuses, containing 200 mg per pill. It was clear that my caffeine intake was far from moderate.

I learned that the effect of caffeine depends on dosage and body weight. Large doses of caffeine can cause altered conscious state, vomiting, abdominal pain, heart arrhythmia, coma, and even death. Lethal doses of caffeine are from five to ten grams. Large doses of caffeine can make the heart race much too fast. The body can even shut down as a protective measure.

Caffeine has been linked to heart disease, benign fibrocystic breast disease, and non-hormone-related breast cancer. Excessive consumption of caffeine by males can cause infertility. For pregnant women, there is the risk of miscarriages, still-births, premature deliveries, and infant deaths.

The most obvious and familiar problem I found about caffeine was that it's a stimulant that disturbs the central nervous system and a strong diuretic; although I didn't know caffeine excretes calcium, magnesium, potassium, folic acid, and vitamin C from the body. I was already convinced I should quit, but I kept reading.

Caffeine stimulates stress hormone production. The jolt we get from caffeine is actually a stress hormone rush. However, the constant artificial cortisol pumping through the use of caffeine exhausts the adrenal glands and leads to their depletion. It affects the proper function of the endocrine, immune, and nervous systems, which may lead to hormonal imbalance, chronic fatigue, fibromyalgia, weight gain, adult onset diabetes, low blood pressure, irritability, anxiety, depression, problems with concentration, sleep disorders, allergies, frequent colds and virus outbreaks, asthma, acute and chronic respiratory and other infections, rhinitis, ulcers, arthritis, decreased thyroid function, ischemic heart disease, hypoglycemia, alcoholism, and even decreased sex drive. Difficult menopause, menstrual cycles (PMS) and altered menstrual flow can definitely be related to adrenal depletion.

I couldn't believe caffeine directly or indirectly can lead to so many health problems. This scary information and my personal problems I had with caffeine left me with no doubts that I had to break my habit.

It was Saturday and finals were coming up Monday. I knew that I shouldn't attempt such a feat before exam week, but a voice inside me kept urging me to try. I don't know where I got the nerve, but I knew I had to do it. I couldn't keep on going the way I was.

Vanity gave me initial strength. My appearance meant a lot to me, but I didn't look my best anymore. My eyes weren't clear. I noticed fine wrinkles at the sides of my eyes and beneath my lower eyelids. I had small pimples across my forehead. My skin was sallow. I could disguise some of the damage, but makeup could not hide chronic fatigue, thinning hair, and a nasty disposition, no matter how carefully it was applied.

I began on Monday morning. I promised myself that I wouldn't touch the 12-packs of Diet Coke beneath my bed. To have them accessible was, for me, part of the exercise in willpower. I also kept them in case the withdrawal symptoms became too great. I expected headaches, and I was not wrong. These headaches had the intensity of migraines.

I lay extremely still in my bed and fell into what seemed to be a sleep coma. When I tried to get up, I felt as though an elephant were standing on my head. Once I got out of bed, I was so lightheaded that I nearly fell. While getting dressed, I kept going into the bed every minute or so to take a short rest break and to lessen the painful grip of the headache.

During the exam, the pain became so awful that I couldn't understand the English language. I had to be excused. I was given one week to complete a make-up exam. I did the same for the rest of my exams and retired to my dorm room for days. It took a while to recover and restore my health to its former pre-caffeine-addicted state.

Chasing academic success had led me to caffeine addiction. Ironically, caffeine nearly destroyed the success I sought. Nothing was worth losing my mental and physical health over. Nothing was worth what I had to go through to break the addiction, and I hope nothing ever will be.

~ 8th Confession ~
Ten Days Between
Hell and Eden

Eighteen years ago I was promoted to the trading room of an investment brokerage firm. If you have seen the movie *Wall Street*, you can picture the crowded trading desks, buzzing computers, and phones ringing nonstop. It is even noisier and more hectic in real life. There were only three other women besides me in this bastion of men. I was young, eager to prove myself, and needed to be "on" from the seven a.m. pre-opening meeting until the four p.m. closing bell.

When you are a trader, you do not leave your desk. You pee in record time, running full speed (in my case, in high heels) to the rest room. Lunches and drinks are brought by a delivery service and paid for by the company. Every fiber of your being is focused on your computers and phones. You are a money machine, and you get paid accordingly.

So how did I keep focused? Caffeine. On my way to work, I fueled myself on a 64-ounce cup of diet cola, which I finished on the commute. At work, I dipped into the refrigerator under my desk at least 12 times per day for a diet cola. I ruined three keyboards in one week as I knocked over my "nectar of the gods." My heart raced, I was hyper, intense, and my temper flared at the slightest provocation because I was over-caffeinated.

I went to school two nights a week to get my MBA. I wanted those coveted letters after my name. After working all day, I endured three-hour classes until nine p.m. I hit the vending machine when I got to class and also at every break, replenishing my rocket fuel.

At night, I rarely slept more than a few hours. I awoke with skull-crushing headaches, easily cured by a can of cola (I usually kept one at my bedside) followed by an Excedrin chaser. I kept a journal by my bed to jot down middle of the night "inspirations," which often resulted in sales memos. I read prospectuses and industry literature, did homework, and was over-prepared for the regular morning meeting. When I had company in bed, orgasms eluded me, as I could never let myself go completely. Each morning, I covered the caffeine hives on my face with makeup and began the cycle again.

I got married. I got pregnant. I cut back on diet cola, but couldn't cut it out. Two of my three children were premature. One of my preemies did not survive.

I had a new activity to occupy my nights, getting up with two babies who were 20 months apart, and caffeine continued to be the mainstay of my diet. To regain my pre-baby figure, I often replaced food with diet cola. As I juggled toddler gym, story time, and play dates, caffeine kept me ready for action.

I could not sleep on my stomach because my cyst-filled breasts were too painful. "Do you drink a lot of caffeine?" my doctor asked me when I went for my annual exam. I wondered how he knew. Weren't breasts supposed to be rock hard?

After seven years at a trading desk, I was promoted to management. I flourished and was happier than I ever was in the trading room. Then the edict came. A conglomerate was acquiring our firm, and I was supposed to run the merger that would put me out of a job. I had to grit my teeth, smile, and pretend I was delighted that these invaders were taking over the firm. I worked 15-hour days until the merger was finished. I worked at home, I worked at the office every day and evening, always accompanied by my loyal friend, diet cola.

Then I became unemployed, something I had not experienced since I was a teenager. I panicked because we had a mortgage, car payments, and other bills. My husband was on disability, so I had to work. We would lose everything if I didn't work. I took two weeks off to be home with my husband and kids, discovered that I was not meant to invade his daytime domain, and went to work in the tech industry. I was delighted to see the subsidized soda machine and free coffee.

I was in a sales position with programmers who were glued to their computer screens. They drank more coffee than the traders ever did. One guy boasted about the calcium deposits he had under his skin from overuse of caffeine. Another demonstrated how his hands shook. Being caffeinated was a badge of honor. The company shut down just a few months later.

I was hired a few weeks later by a more established tech company, which had an even stronger culture of coffee and cola. These programmers built custom programs for state and local governments on tight deadlines. For added pleasure, energy drinks containing multiple times the caffeine of coffee or soda were thrown back like shots at happy hour.

I learned after a few months that the owner was interested in selling the company and wanted my expertise in sales, networking, and mergers. I spent many caffeine-fueled hours setting things up, now with a new penchant for energy drinks. I replaced my usual glass of chardonnay with a vodka and energy drink cocktail, a souvenir of my tech career.

After this, I went back to what I knew—the investment industry—and became a stockbroker. This happened during a recession. It was hard to find clients, and I was doing commission-only work. My husband did not understand the sudden change in our income. Our marriage was unraveling, and I spent more time away from him, taking the kids on weekend outings and doing all I could to avoid him. I sought comfort with my soda. Caffeine kept me awake, so I would not have to get into the bed next to my new enemy. Instead, I stayed up to read and watch television.

We separated, and I landed an investment management job at another firm, this time with a salary and bonus structure. I was better able to support my kids and myself, and pay for the attorney for my divorce.

Fueled on caffeine, I was wired during the depositions, ready to jump at my attacker. I nearly leapt over the table in court at him as he told bald-faced lies. However, I took my attorney team's advice and maintained a placid expression, despite biting my cheeks until they bled. I got the house, the kids, and child support.

I dated a series of men, each one more narcissistic and wired than the next. Then I met the One. He was like no one I had ever met before. He had been to over 300 Grateful Dead shows, which I thought was a cool accomplishment. He maintained a healthy diet and did not consume caffeine. He liked music, skiing, bike riding, snowshoeing, nature walks, and golf, and introduced me to these things as well. He liked going out to dinner and talking about subjects that mattered, even though he was quiet by nature. He loved hanging out with my kids and pets. I continued to be my caffeinated self, and he never asked me to change. One of his first gifts to me was a bar of caffeinated soap. I was hooked on him after that.

Suddenly, one afternoon, my body was wracked in pain. I was feverish and could not keep anything down, not even diet cola. In a matter of hours, I was bedridden with the worst flu I have ever had in my life. For three days I sipped ginger ale and ate crackers. I had no diet cola in the house. I wanted to pick some up, but was too ill. My illness was compounded by tremendous headaches, hand tremors, and lethargy. I felt confused and anxious. By the time I was over the flu, I had gone without caffeine for days.

When I slept I had dreams, something that had not happened in years. The headaches slowly abated, and my skin started to clear from its ever-present redness. I was extremely thirsty and consumed large amount of water and sodium-free seltzer. I couldn't seem to quench my thirst.

I decided I would give up caffeine since the worst part of the withdrawal appeared to be over. I needed a substitute for my oral fixation and found solace with ice water and seltzer. I was tempted to fall back into my diet cola ways as my body still craved it, but I stuck to my guns. I realize now that I was giving up two foreign substances, caffeine and Nutrasweet. My withdrawal symptoms spoke loud and clear. It took about ten days before I felt normal, with no headaches, anxiety, cravings, and irritability.

One thing I discovered is that water is widely accessible and very en vogue. It's available at parties, coffee shops, people's homes, restaurants, bars, hotels, and anywhere else, even in vending machines.

Nobody has ever made a negative comment about my "sparkling water with lime" drink order or when I am sipping bottled water at my desk. I drink at least eight glasses of water per day, just as medical wisdom has dictated for years.

Now, a year later, I have flawless skin, have lost weight, am calmer, less irritable, sleep well at night—even on my stomach—and am full of energy. A morning walk around the block wakes me up just as much as caffeine once did. I enjoy my children more, and I am a better mom because I am less frazzled. I am still a high performer at work, motivated by challenge rather than stimulants. People comment on how youthful I look, thinking I am younger than 43. Best of all, my sex life is better than ever —"O" does not just stand for Oprah!

I am still with the One. It's been over five years now. He loves the new and improved me. He says that I am more fun, sexier, and less intense than when he first met me. We recently flew across the country, and he said that in the past he would worry that I would nervously chatter nonstop on the flight. Instead, I read a book, slept, and chatted calmly and pleasantly.

I feel healthier, happier, and smarter than ever before and ready to face whatever life sends my way.

~ 9th Confession ~
The Society Trap

I never thought I had a problem. I mean, you read about every kind of addict: alcohol, drugs, or sex. I used to flip through magazines reading about people who suffered from addiction and how they lost everything—family, friends, and jobs. I read these stories while sipping my morning coffee and thinking how lucky I was to be so grounded. By my fifth cup of coffee, I would have read the entire magazine.

I felt destined to be a teacher. I had received high marks at the university, and by the time I started my student teaching, I was ready to make a difference. Everything I had learned—the philosophy of teaching, methods, cognitive development, and classroom management—were all at the forefront of my mind. However, you could never be ready for what is thrown at you.

My first week in school was a nightmare. On the first day, my mentor was so busy that she didn't even have time to introduce herself. By day two, she was absent, and I was thrown into full swing. By the third day, I was trapped after class by an angry parent. Apparently, I had greatly hurt the feelings of a child whom I had called by the wrong name. After I spent almost an hour trying to apologize, the woman left when she realized she was late for a meeting.

I turned around to face the empty classroom. Books were scattered across the floor, a bottle of glue had spilled all over the rug, and on my desk was a sea of ungraded papers, letters from parents, and a memo reminding me that I was supposed to be at a teacher's meeting an hour ago. When I took off down the hallway, the teachers were leaving the meeting. My mentor saw me and asked in a stern voice where I had been. That's when I lost it. The tears welled up. I flew back into my classroom and buried my head in shame.

My mentor came in and closed the door behind her. I felt the calming touch of her hand on my back. "So," she said, "your first week hasn't turned out to be quite what you were expecting."

I just nodded, as it was all I could do.

"My name's Janice, by the way. Janice Anderson," she said. "Why don't I get us both a fresh cup of coffee, and then we can get to know each other."

I never drank coffee. I tried once, but I hated the taste and felt hyper and nervous afterward. But at that moment, with my shirt stained with tears and the events of the previous days still coursing through my veins, it sounded wonderful. Mrs. Anderson brought two large cups of coffee back into our untidy classroom. With the first sip, I felt better.

We talked for over an hour. She listened with empathy while I talked about feeling lost in the classroom. When I began to tell her about the angry parent, she insisted we have another cup and we went to the teachers' lounge. "Angry parents are the worst, but they are sadly a reality of teaching that we all have to face," she said. Other teachers overheard what we were talking about, and they all came into the room with cups of coffee to exchange war stories. By the end of it all, I had met all the teachers and the principal, and I was feeling much more welcome.

I used the weekend to rest, reflect, and move on. On Monday, I arrived at school on time for the morning meeting. Mrs.

Anderson sat next to me to discuss the week's lessons. When the school secretary passed around coffee, I didn't really want it, but I thanked her and drank my cup.

My second week was slightly smoother. Mrs. Anderson put me in charge of reading, math, and science. "You need to develop a three-week plan for math and science for kindergarten and first grade, and include modifications for all 'learner differences,'" she said. I nodded, writing this down for my weekend to-do list. "You need this by tomorrow," she added.

I stayed after school that night and worked until I had finished everything. By ten p.m. I had fallen asleep on my desk. On Friday, I was dragging myself through each hour, and when the kids were on the bus, papers were graded, and the meeting adjourned, there was Mrs. Anderson with coffee. I sat down with her again, feeling much more confident than the week before.

The weeks continued, with road bumps, small victories, and an occasional angry parent. All the while, coffee was part of it all. I guess I had acquired a taste for it. It became essential to have coffee every morning at school. I started to feel groggy in the mornings, which was strange for me because I had always been a morning person. The school cup of coffee went from being something that I participated in if offered to something that I depended on. The school week was very hectic and filled with many coffee breaks. For a while, coffee was still something I associated with school. I didn't have any at home since my mom thought it was poison, and my friends never drank any either.

The first sign of addiction came when I had to go without coffee. I rode my bike to school one Monday morning to discover that Mrs. Anderson was ill and I would be taking over the class. My initial instinct was to grab a cup of coffee. I started to walk towards the teachers' room when the second grade teacher came running up. "Can you stay here with Robert? He came early today, and I have to meet with a parent." Before I had even agreed to do it, she was out of sight.

I had a surge of panic, thinking about all the things I had to do. I saw the school lunch lady smoking outside and managed to get her attention. She wasn't happy about staying with Robert, but she agreed. The smell of coffee from the teachers' room worked like a jolt to my system, and I again headed that way, but the phone in my classroom started ringing. Mrs. Anderson had been very clear about the importance of answering the phone at all times. She had explained to me that usually only parents and teachers would call the classroom, and so we should always stop anything to answer the phone. So I did. It was a parent—an angry parent. The reason for her anger isn't important, but she was angry and she yelled. Twenty minutes passed, and she was still yelling. Teachers came in and out wanting to talk. Parents lined up wanting to talk to me. I couldn't get off the phone. When the kids started flooding into the room, I had to interrupt her and end the call. The clock was already ten minutes past the time we normally began lessons, and the kids were running all over the room. Finally, after the last parent left, I slammed the door and yelled loudly at the kids to sit down. They all stopped and stared at me stone-faced. I had never yelled like that before. I didn't care. We had so much to do and my head was pounding. The day didn't get any better. If the kids asked for help, I told them to sit down and keep trying.

At the end of the day, I went to the teachers' lounge only to find there was no more coffee. I was infuriated. I felt like they had planned it. I honestly imagined smacking the next person who approached me, but I didn't. I took a walk down the street to Starbucks. The only thought I had was to get my hands on the largest cup of coffee I could find. The smell inside the Starbucks was exhilarating. The menu had flavors and options that I hadn't even known existed. I ordered an extra tall cappuccino with extra sugar. With every sip my problems seemed to melt away. I got out a novel that I had been dying to read, but couldn't because of work. I sat there and read the first six chapters and then ordered another cappuccino and a piece of chocolate cake. I began to go to Starbucks every day after school and read there for hours. At the end of my student teaching, I had stopped giving 110 percent at school. I soon said goodbye to my students and Mrs. Anderson. I was going to miss them, but I felt good about moving on.

I decided to take a few weeks off before starting to look for jobs. I spent a lot of time at Starbucks catching up on all the reading I had missed during the student teaching. I started smoking, something I had sworn never to do, but only when leaving Starbucks.

When a few weeks out of work became a few months, my mom started to nag at me. She had agreed to let me live with her while I did student teaching, but she thought it was unhealthy for me to be freeloading any longer. She continually asked when I was going to find a job, why I was looking so unhealthy, and whether I was smoking. I finally snapped at her and stormed out of the house with a pounding head-ache, mad at the world. I drove to Starbucks that day; it seemed too far to go by bike. Inside, I stood fidgeting, glaring at everyone else in line. I wanted to push them out of the way when they couldn't decide what to order. When it was finally my turn, I snapped at the girl behind the register, "Give me an extra large coffee!"

"What kind of coffee would you like?" she asked.

I lost my patience and barked, "Just give me a coffee!"

I grabbed the coffee and stormed out. I drove around looking for another Starbucks. When I found one, I was slightly calmer and went through three more cups. I was so wired and nervous that I could barely drive home.

I was up to about three pots of coffee a day. I started keeping coffee at home, even though my mom wasn't happy about that and was already starting to comment on the new yellowish glow on my teeth.

The mood swings continued. I couldn't feel motivated to look for a real job. I took a part-time job in a bookstore instead. I spent my days driving to work, drinking coffee, and reading. The pay was awful, but I made enough to support my habits. I use the plural because I was now smoking regularly. My friends had all started real jobs. I didn't care. I would just drink coffee and laugh at it all. I could vent to the middle-aged hippies I worked with and the high school kids who came in after school. We would drink coffee together and fill each other's heads with plans for the future. I'd often babble about the stories I would write.

I'd tell myself that I'd go home and start writing, but it never happened. I'd go home to an angry mother who wondered what had happened to my teaching career. It was none of her business, I'd say. By the time I would sit down to write I was too fidgety, and my head would swim with incomprehensible thoughts. I finally decided to see the doctor.

Dr. H. had treated me my entire life. He said that the last time he saw me I was studying to be a teacher. When he said this, my heart kind of sank. I hoped that he wouldn't ask what I was doing now, but of course he did. I lied. I told him I was working as a reading specialist. I couldn't bring myself to admit the truth.

He asked the usual questions and gave me a full exam. He asked if I give myself regular breast exams, and I said no. He said I needed to be sure to check myself every month. As he checked my breasts, he asked if I had been consuming an unusual amount of caffeine. I thought it was an odd question.

"Well, just a few cups," I said. "I guess about three cups in the morning, then one for the road…one to start the day at work, then several coffee breaks...a couple of cups after lunch, and then one on the way home. I usually make an after-dinner pot, but that's about it." I wanted him to tell me that it was normal. I don't know why, but for the first time since I started drinking coffee, I felt really ashamed.

He grabbed my hand and placed it on my breast. "Do you feel these lumps?"

"Yes," I said. There were too many to count.

"They are not cancerous, but you are far from healthy," he said. "These lumps are the result of an overconsumption of the drug caffeine."

It was the first time that I heard the word "drug" used to refer to caffeine.

He continued to question me: Did I suffer from mood swings? Yes. Did I suffer from headaches? Yes, all the time. Did I suffer from feelings of lethargy? Yes, all the time. Did I find it hard to concentrate, feel fidgety, or suffer from a short temper? Yes. Yes. Yes!

By the end of the visit, Dr. H. had officially diagnosed me with an addiction to caffeine. His advice was to reduce to one or two cups a day if I had to have some. The cigarettes had to go.

I felt as if I had been hit by a truck. Couldn't he just write out a prescription and be done with it? Wasn't there some sort of magical cure to bring me back to where I was before the student teaching? I could live without coffee. How did I get into this mess in the first place? I told myself that it wasn't a big deal. After all, until that visit, I never really felt that I had a problem. On the drive home, I got out a cigarette, lit up, and started puffing away while I pulled into the first Starbucks I saw. I ordered my usual, and it hit me: I didn't really want coffee. I hadn't even thought about it. It was just a habit. My heart sank again, as I realized that I was an addict.

I didn't want my mom to know what the doctor had said. I could quit. Just thinking about it made me happy. I was so high on this idea that I wanted to make a pot of coffee. I would quit the next day.

The next day I didn't have to work. I could sleep in and then go for a bike ride. It had been so long since I had ridden my bike. I looked in the mirror. I had put on weight. Lost muscle tone. This made me feel very low. Downstairs I got the coffee out, ready to make a pot. Then it hit me, "Today is my quitting day." I went out to get my bike. The tires were flat. I pumped up the tires and took off. After ten minutes, I felt a burning sensation in my lungs. I caught my breath and started out again, but I felt bad. My head started to pound. I passed a Starbucks and smelled the intoxicating aroma. I couldn't resist. I walked inside and ordered the usual. After three of the usual my headache was gone. I cycled home and watched television.

By dinner I couldn't take it, and so I made coffee. It was official. I had a problem. I decided to confess to my mom what the doctor had told me. I told her everything that was on my mind. I told her how I felt angry all the time, and tired, and physically ill. All the while, she listened patiently. She didn't nag or say that she told me so. She made me a cup of herbal tea, caffeine-free, and we drank tea together. In that moment she reminded me of Mrs. Anderson during that first week of student teaching. I remembered how good it felt to have someone wiser listen with an open mind. Then I started to talk openly to my mom about where I began to go wrong. It was clear that I needed to change direction. I needed to get healthy again.

I gave up coffee and cigarettes. It wasn't easy. It took the help of everyone around me. I started to research caffeine addiction. I read up on what caffeine had been doing to my body and mind. I gave myself reasonable benchmarks. For the first month, I could have three cups a day. When I wanted more, I either drank water or went for a bike ride. Sometimes I did both. By month two I had cut out the after-dinner coffee. That was hard. I had to switch to caffeine-free herbal tea and water. Coffee slowly became something I could control, as opposed to something that controlled me. What I really had to examine was my emotional dependence on caffeine. I had grown to rely on it as a crutch. I needed an alternative method for dealing with stress. I thought about my mom and Mrs. Anderson. They had both helped me through critical points in my life. My weakness led me to addiction; my strength led me to recovery.

~ 10th Confession ~
Writer's Block

I tried to quit caffeine a few times. I'm not exactly Batman in the willpower department, but my biggest problem was I thought I couldn't write without caffeine.

At first I wanted to quit because a four-dollar cup of coffee every morning was killing my wallet. A large cup of coffee with a shot of espresso from Dunkin' Donuts comes to around three dollars. With tip, I was spending about 112 dollars per month, so I stopped buying it. The first day I felt dizzy, tired and achy, but I figured it was probably a bad night's sleep. The second day, putting inventory on shelves at work hurt my arms, I had trouble walking in a straight line, and my vision seemed limited to a thin cone. The headaches alone would have kept a weaker man home. It took me a while to figure out that the problem was caffeine. I made it to my lunch break and ran to the nearby Dunkin' Donuts, which made everything better.

My friends, my girlfriend, and I would usually go to Denny's on Wednesday, after we got paid. Okay, almost any night was Denny's. We would get drinks and fries and hang around for hours, doing different things: My friends drew, I wrote, and my girlfriend would admire my friends' art and my writing. Our waiter, Glen, knew our drink orders by heart: three of us had coffee and one had tea. Somewhere between my fourth and eighth cup of coffee I would pull out a legal pad and write about my day. When I skipped the coffee, my friends rated my writing as somewhere between "unnerving" and "get help."

Around during the second time I tried to quit, on the second night, I was on my way to Denny's where I was meeting more than the usual crowd. A couple of my other friends were there, including a few of those whom I didn't talk to anymore. When my girlfriend and I sat down, Glen came over and confirmed our usual order, "Coffee and coffee, right?"

"Actually, could I get a hot chocolate?" I asked. The caffeine content was low, and it was the only other hot drink with free refills. The table was more silent than it probably should have been.

"What's the matter," said Glen, "our coffee's not good enough for you?"

"Yeah, dude, what the hell," said one of my friends.

Others were more malicious. It's not like they were saying anything different, but there was a definite difference in their tone. I was the target of their jokes for disrupting the status quo that night. The jokes were cruel. I had a headache from caffeine withdrawal, felt groggy, and wasn't in the mood to put up with it. I left early that night.

When I arrived home, I researched as much as I could about caffeine, caffeine addiction, and its side effects. I learned all sorts of statistics: when a caffeine high peaks, how long it lasts, how much caffeine was in my morning coffee, and how much it takes to create a physical addiction. I also learned that withdrawal peaked at about 48 hours.

That explained why the second day had been so bad. Armed with an arsenal of data, I resolved to quit not for my wallet but for my health.

I lasted about three days. It wasn't the headaches or the disorientation that got to me, though they didn't do me any good. On the third day, I opened a blank document and put my hands on the keyboard—and that was as far as I got. I couldn't write. The cursor was blinking as if to say, "Feed me, feed me with your words..." I made a pot of coffee.

It was another few months before I tried to quit coffee again.

Money had again gotten tight, and I was looking for things I could cut out of my budget. Coffee seemed an obvious choice, but the memory of that blank monitor always came back. My girlfriend reminded me of my favorite nonfiction book, Stephen King's memoirs *On Writing*. In it he discusses, among other topics, his addiction to cocaine and how he once thought he couldn't write without getting high. Keeping that in mind, I shamed myself into quitting. Stephen King got over cocaine addiction. I drank coffee.

I did a lot of reading about how to quit drugs. One bit of advice was to tell friends what you're doing, so I explained to my friends that I was going to quit caffeine. One friend told me I was pathetic because I couldn't handle caffeine. Another said it wasn't even worth trying. The third said I wouldn't be allowed in his house because he didn't want to deal with me moping around. My close friends, the Denny's group, were completely supportive, barring the occasional snide joke.

I went about a month without writing anything. I tried a few times, but it was painful. I'd sit at my computer, staring at the screen. I'd write a sentence, "So there's this guy..." and I'd know it was drivel. Not only was it drivel, but I didn't know what came next. I'd write scraps of a story with no plot, or I'd outline a plot and be unable to write the story. Every time I'd write, I'd think about having a cup of coffee. I finally stopped writing until my body got used to not having caffeine.

Then one day I got some lines in my head. They were the first few words of a poem. I wrote them out. I came up with a few more lines. I edited the first ones, and then wrote more until there was a poem in front of me. It was almost good. I started to write more poems. I'd write two or three poems in an hour. Usually one of them was good. It was like high. I was getting giddy. I'd call it the most rewarding experience of my life.

It's been about four months since I quit caffeine. I've written three short stories, a number of poems, and have gone back to work on my novel. I write every day now. It's fantastic. I'm doing better financially, but the extra 100 dollars a month I'm saving doesn't hurt. The only problem is avoiding thoughts like "just one cup." Furthermore, I feel better physically. I'm not dizzy in the morning and getting out of bed has become easier.

I used to believe that people weren't able to think well without caffeine or some other drug. However, I've proven myself wrong. I'm much more capable now without headaches and dehydration from caffeine. It feels as if a weight has been lifted from my mind. I'm also not triggered by the wired people with whom I converse. I've only been caffeine-free for a few months, but I really think I've quit for life.

~ 11th Confession ~
Devil's Chemical

During my junior year at high school, I started using caffeine tablets. I needed to stay focused, so I could pass my SATs. I had no intention of staying on them after the SATs. Unaware of how addicting these tablets were, I used them daily. I had a weekend job, so I could buy them without my mother's knowledge. After school, I hung out with my boyfriend, Derryck, or with friends. When I got home at night, I took a caffeine tablet and began studying. Sleep was not a significant factor. I allowed myself only four hours of sleep. In the morning I took another tablet to stay focused in school. Fridays, I went out with Derryck and friends. Saturdays, I always had a hangover and slept until the afternoon. Then I went to my job at Kroger. Sundays, I got up early to go to work again. I usually worked overtime since I needed the money. Caffeine tablets are not cheap, but I felt I needed them to do well in school. I did not realize I had become addicted.

The night before the SATs, I stayed home studying. I took four caffeine tablets and didn't sleep at all. When it came time to go to school, I took two more tablets. I was jumpy, shaky, but awake. During the second hour of the test I couldn't focus or keep still. The proctor asked me if I was okay. I told him I was just a little nervous. When the third hour rolled around, I could not focus well enough to answer the questions.

The test was over, but I still kept taking the tablets. I also began to drink coffee every morning, during breaks in school, and each afternoon. By now, my mom noticed a change in my attitude and behavior.

She thought I had a drug problem. I couldn't deny it without admitting my addiction to caffeine. So I played along and went to drug addiction meetings. I was still taking caffeine tablets, but it was less noticeable because I avoided my house as much as I could. I would stay out all day and come home at night. My mom worked night shifts, so it was easy to avoid her. I also took more shifts at work, partly so I could afford my tablets. I got Derryck addicted to caffeine as well. It felt good to be able to share my secret with someone. He was unemployed, so I was paying for his addiction, too. During the summer after my junior year, I tried to quit. I couldn't.

Summer was over, and I wanted to buckle down and do well. Although I was still under the influence of caffeine, I was improving my grades, getting all A's and B's. I wanted to go to college, and my grades were very important to me. I made friends with exchange students and that improved my French. My mom and verbally abusive stepdad divorced, but he still lived with us. This was one of the reasons I did not want to be home at all. I spent most of my time at the house of a new friend. Sometimes I stayed in Derryck's apartment.

Then things started falling apart. My mom and stepdad remarried, and he started acting like my "guardian" again. To avoid him, I was always at my friend's house. But after learning about my caffeine addiction, she began to avoid me. Derryck's apartment was always open, but I did not like his place. So I had to stay at home. Mom was delighted, but I was not. I stayed in my room most of the time, trying to avoid comments about my behavior and questions about my problems. My sleep disorder was one. I woke up many times during the night. I went for one evening without taking any tablets, but woke up with nightmares.

70

I could not stop taking the caffeine tablets. Even if I had enough strength, Derryck would never have let me. He appeared to have become more addicted than I was. He came to my house daily to ask for more tablets. I'd give them to him willingly because he was the only person who shared my addiction.

I found an inexpensive way to feed my addiction. I'd buy Folgers. My mom, she got the whole month off from her job and was always at home, noticed how much coffee I was drinking. I'd come downstairs at least ten times a day to fill my coffee mug. I started having panic attacks. I did not know I was suffering from an anxiety disorder related to my caffeine intake. My mom was concerned about my coffee addiction. She also found caffeine tablets in my room. I knew I should be prepared for some sort of intervention from my family.

One day when Derryck drove me home from school, I saw my stepfather's sedan in the driveway. The only reasons I could think of why he would be home at this hour were that either he had been fired or that he was preparing for the ambush I was expecting. I told Derryck I wanted to go to his apartment. I stayed for two nights. When I got home, my stepdad was lying on the couch. He had been diagnosed with prostate cancer. Since the cancer was detected early, he should be okay. I thought his diagnosis would take the focus off my addiction.

However, two days later, my mom cornered me while I was getting my third cup of coffee. After a brutal argument, I left. I wasn't planning to return. I stayed with Derryck through the end of high school. I made it into a local college, but rarely attended classes. I was still taking caffeine tablets. My poor work habits finally got me fired from Kroger, so I went to work at Burger King.

A year after high school, I got pregnant. I knew large doses of caffeine could be dangerous for a baby, but I didn't know how to quit. I had been on caffeine tablets daily for over three years. I

71

still was as immature as I had been in high school, but Derryck had moved on. He wanted a baby, so he gave me ultimatum: Stop taking caffeine tablets or he would leave me. I loved Derryck, but somehow caffeine meant more to me. I could imagine my life without Derryck, but not without caffeine tablets. However, I couldn't raise a baby alone, and I was raised to be against abortion. I told him I would quit, but I couldn't.

One day he caught me with the tablets. We had a fight, and he tried to grab my tablets. I don't know why, but I simply couldn't give them to him. I gripped the vial in my fist as tightly as I could. His face changed. Overwhelmed with rage, he said exactly what he thought of me. Everything was over between us.

Luckily, my mom had left her door open. I went to live with her, but I did not stay long. During the first trimester, I had a miscarriage. In a way, I was relieved. I couldn't take care of a baby. I couldn't even take care of myself.

The miscarriage transformed me. It became clear I had to make serious changes in my life in order to move forward. I began attending Narcotics Anonymous meetings. At first, when I explained that my drug of choice was caffeine, the others made jokes. To this day, it is hard for people to believe that caffeine is a drug. I kept going to the meetings anyway, and they stopped joking. I am back in school now. I live with my new boyfriend and frequently visit my mom. Her support helped pull me through.

~ 12th Confession ~
Quantum of Solace

The silence of the empty newsroom engulfs me. Not a soul around except for the night shift producer, who, in a state of drowsiness, is gradually passing out on his chair. It's 1:40 a.m. I still have to finish my script and then edit my story.

I take a sip of coffee, finish my script, and run toward the edit bay. I hand my work to my editor and head back to my desk. My coffee has gone cold. I go to the pantry to make another cup to help me stay awake during long working hours.

My caffeine addiction started in journalism school, when assignments, research papers, and book reviews kept me up until the wee hours of the morning. My best friend became a mug of black coffee. A shot of espresso and I was set for two hours of nonstop study.

Multiple assignments led to continuous sleepless nights, and I added energy drinks. When I finally tried to sleep, I couldn't because my brain was so wired that it refused to rest. Those times were nightmarish. It did not dawn upon me exactly what I was doing and how it would affect me eventually.

After journalism school, I started to work. From breaking news to running after exclusives, life as a reporter was always on the edge. The competition between who gets the news first is fierce. The frustration and stress led to a greater dependence on stimulants. I went from one cigarette to a pack and replaced water with coffee. I had to be mentally alert all the time. One slack moment and I could miss an important detail or piece of information, which could cost me my job. And in such a business you can eschew mental peace, but not on an important piece of news.

Sleep deprivation caused dark circles under my eyes. The loss of appetite from excessive consumption of caffeine affected me both internally and externally. The worst effect of my addiction came as a blow to me the day I realized that I had lost myself in it. I had lost my peace of mind. I was not the old me anymore. I would get ticked off at the slightest provocation. I had mood swings and felt edgy most of the time. The lack of sleep and loss of appetite added to my stress.

I was dating a guy I had known for three years. My increasing career responsibilities did not leave time to see him anymore. The problems between us kept increasing. The tension led to fights. I could not control myself and would lose my temper. My anxiety and agitation made me feel negative about everything around me. He insisted that I had become a changed person and was not the girl he had loved.

Maybe I knew it myself, but when it came from the person with whom I had imagined spending a lifetime, it crushed my spirit. I thought our relationship was the root of my anxiety and that ending it would eliminate my stress. Thus I broke up with the man I had believed I would marry. The solace had come from work as I drowned myself in assignments. I was so involved with my career that everything else seemed frivolous. I had stopped having a life of my own.

Then I took on an assignment that required three days of rigorous shooting. At the end of the third day, I collapsed. I was rushed to the hospital and diagnosed with colitis. I was hospitalized for three weeks. Lack of proper food and excessive consumption of caffeine on an empty stomach had ruined my digestive system.

I had no one. I chose not to contact my family, who lived miles away. My friends had disappeared because of my lack of communication. I had broken up with my boyfriend. Lying on the hospital bed with not a soul around, I knew I had to make a new start.

During those three weeks in the hospital, I read Sylvia Plath's The Bell Jar, a dark, brooding tale of a girl suffering from neurosis. The idea that sleep deprivation could result in neurosis scared the daylights out of me. Additional reading made me aware that regular sleep is important for health. I read more about how to prepare for sleep by taking a shower, having a mild drink, or listening to soft music to soothe the nerves.

When I went back to work after a month's rest, a lot had changed in me. I realized that in the quest for fame and recognition I was slowly losing myself. I could not afford to do that anymore. The first step I took was asking my boss to shift me to the desk. I realized that I could not handle the pressures of working as a field reporter. The next step was the Art of Living course, which combined yoga with meditation and a healthy lifestyle. Next, I reduced my caffeine intake. I could not cut it out completely.

I still take my morning cup of black coffee, but now I eat something with it. During the day I have replaced coffee with herbal tea. I do not take caffeine in any form in the evening. I have reduced smoking and eat four to five small meals a day. I have learned to be happy and take things much more lightly than I used to because, at the end of the day, it's your mental peace that will ultimately help you go places. In the never-ending race of life, at times we forget exactly for what and for whom we are taking all the trouble.

I know now that that magic potion, caffeine, can seem to be the solution to problems, but its long-term effects are nothing less than scary. The tricky part of caffeine addiction is that you do not even realize when it has turned into a problem. It starts as a lifestyle norm and slowly takes over as an integral part of your existence. The influence of this evil in disguise takes a while to recognize. I found my way out only when I had no other option.

~ 13th Confession ~
Her Name Was Caffeine

Caffeine is a gorgeous demon with vibrant hair, warm skin, and wide eyes burning with ambition. I was snagged by those fishhook lips and knew pulling away would be painful. I gave my academic life, social life, love life, and body to that vile seductress. At first, it was harmonious. Then I needed her, and soon I became dependent.

High school was the most difficult time of my life. Staying conscious through calculus at eight a.m. was quite a feat. I was struggling. My grades were slipping. The teachers were soulless. The school was originally built to be a prison and had no windows. I was empty. I needed something. Then one day a big, beautiful blue truck pulled up to my school. The driver unloaded several humming, glowing vending machines.

The next day, about an hour before calculus, I purchased a 20-ounce bottle of Mountain Dew. By the time calculus rolled around, something was different: I was awake! I could focus, converse, and not feel completely dreadful. My transformation was so noticeable that it prompted a friend to ask, "Did you meet a girl or something? You're more alive than usual, especially for calc class." In fact, I had met a girl. Her name was Caffeine.

Everyday before calculus she was waiting for me. My grades began to ascend, and my social life began to improve. Then one day, after a particularly late night, I forgot my dollar twenty-five.

During calculus, not only was I battling a severe sandman onslaught, but I had one of the most skull-grating headaches I have ever experienced. The drowsiness and headaches continued throughout that terrible day. I vowed that I wouldn't go another day without my dose. I bought a pack of 24 Mountain Dews.

That night a friend came over and by morning the box was empty. Twelve cans apiece, 144 ounces each. That's too much. I didn't sleep for the rest of the weekend. My friend, on the contrary, did. We attempted to wake him up, but his body refused. We learned later that he experienced a diabetic coma. He awoke, luckily, on Monday. It took him a week or so to finally recover. That was the only warning sign he needed, but not me.

After I told the tale of my sleepless weekend, a few friends and I wanted to see just how far we could go. We were going to stay up for as long as we could. Keeping in mind that the average person could die after ten days without rest, we were searching for a near-death experience.

During the first night, we mixed cocktails of every local and imported energy drink known. We would slam the mixtures, wait until they were absorbed into the bloodstream, then eat and eat and eat. One friend received a concussion after a head injury on a trampoline, but he never complained of any pain. I got a nosebleed after landing face-first on a friend's knee while attempting a somersault. I remember laughing and bleeding, but no pain.

Day two: A "dolphin brain" effect kicked in. Dolphins have the ability to put one half of their brain to sleep, which is what our brains tried to do. The frontal lobe—basically the brain's filter— went to sleep. Our senses became vivid. We were seeing and hearing everything at the same time. We began saying things we didn't know we were saying.

We were drooling and shivering. Our body heat fled; we were always cold.

Day three: The perspective of time vanished. This made it difficult for us to determine how long day three lasted. We stopped being goofy. We couldn't form a cohesive thought. We weren't sure why we couldn't go to sleep, but we couldn't. We decided not to drive anywhere; although no major accidents had occurred, we didn't want to risk it.

Day four: I experienced "sleep deafness." I would nod off in such a way that I wasn't truly asleep. Whether I dozed off for a couple minutes, or slipped into a 14-hour mini-coma, I did not get enough sleep. Another phenomenon is memories. When you sleep, your memory gets a chance to refresh itself. Our memories were overloaded and worthless. We simply could not function.

For me, this is what high school was like. Day by day, caffeine consumed my life. I even wrote lyrics to a song that demonstrated this:

"All Night"

One mocha and I fell in love
Two French vanilla turtledoves cinnamon and hazelnut
cappuccino
Frappuccino
Irish Crème I'll tell you what
Red Bull and a Double Shot
My veins are charged, my head is hot
Amp, Monster, Jolt, Full Throttle
Concoctions of cranial catastrophes
Caffeine capsules by the bottle
Jumping, screaming, burning, spinning
Kamikaze curse beginning
Grizzly-slamming, buckteeth-bashing
Shovel-swinging, sternum-twisting

Artillery in my arteries thrashing
Awake are we, scabs in our hair
Awake are we, and if we dare
We'll never let our unrest break
Awake are we,
Awake are we
Awake, are we awake?

The first year of college was similar to my high school years. Time passed harmoniously with Caffeine brightly buzzing along in the background, but not interfering, so it seemed. I met a beautiful girl. The love between us grew and we wished to have children. So we tried, but failed. My sperm count had plummeted, and my sex-drive was reduced.

I could no longer focus in class. I could no longer play more than five minutes of any sport. Sleep was out of the question. I couldn't love whom I wanted to love. My heart couldn't take it. People forget that caffeine is indeed a drug. It plays by its own rules. It's uncontrollable, and if you don't stop it, it will never be stopped.

By the time I decided to pull the caffeine hooks out, I was consuming 100 ounces or more of energy drinks per day. When you're trying to pull a hook out, there are no painless ways of doing it. But there are smart ways, and one way is to pace yourself. Week by week I dropped ten ounces, then ten more. By the third month, I had debilitating headaches.

I couldn't continue without help. I needed friends to tell me I could succeed, keep me accountable, and rebuild me. Also, I discovered less detrimental ways to get energy. Dr. Pinkus pills, Bumble Bars, and even natural sunlight helped. The most important ingredients in my recipe for recovery were self-discipline and prayer.

Caffeine was a subtle enemy. I wasn't aware that I was under attack, and by the time I noticed, I convinced myself I was gaining more than I was losing. She seemed to be so much help. She only wanted a little from me, then a little more every time after that, until she had everything, until my heart, body, and self-worth were broken. I had a secret weapon, however. I had hope, and that is exactly what it took to turn me around.

Success was sweet. Now my sources of energy are the food I eat, the people I'm around, music, and the sunlight. My sleep cycles are still disrupted, but I am going to be a father this June. Right now Lady Caffeine has her hooks only on my past. My future is bright, beautiful, and—thank God—caffeine-free.

~ 14th Confession ~
With the Help of the Stars

"You have a Pisces moon; you absorb information by osmosis," said my mother, who likes to explain everything in terms of astrology. Had the stars doomed me to become addicted to caffeine?

My father, a lawyer, had the same astrological pronouncements as I did. He stayed up late at night to work because he could not concentrate in his busy daytime office. He said that when he looked at the cases, the words would swim and he would circle them around and around in his head, trying to figure them out. Although he saw different sides of the case and all the details, he could never get to the heart of the matter; his was a diffuse sort of reasoning.

Perhaps it was because he drank too much coffee. Every morning, before anything else, he would set the percolator gurgling. Cold, half-drunk cups curdled in the armrests of the car or turned black on his desk, leaving brown stains on the legal paper. He drank caffeinated soda, too. The kitchen sheltered a refrigerator stocked with rows of diet Coca-Cola, bought wholesale in crates of 100 cans.

When we went to Starbucks, my mother would scan the shelves for collectible merchandise. When Starbucks created souvenir mugs for each major city, my mom claimed Boston,

Houston, and San Francisco. I provided the London mug when I studied there.

As for me, I never liked coffee—burnt acorns, regardless of what kind of mug it was in. It reminded me in taste, texture, and consistency of mud. However, when the stress of academics hit me in college, I remembered that my father always drank coffee, so I thought I would try it. Looking to save my midterm grades, I took my first swig.

After gradually developing a taste for coffee, heavily watered down with cream and sugar, the addictive nature of the substance itself won me over. My addiction intensified. The school system in London required a level of rigor to which I was unaccustomed. I was concerned about making the grade. I also found myself isolated by the way I looked and talked; my American ways were neither appreciated nor tolerated. Being alone in a foreign country caused me to become profoundly homesick. As a result, I found myself craving a sugary treat to go with that simmering brew that provided comfort. Toast and jam? Sure. Nutella? Even better. A slice of chocolate cake? Bring it on. Not only did I crave coffee, but also energy drinks, although I never had before.

I had a coffee ritual during my all-night-studing routine. In a fit of procrastination, I would get what I thought of as a motivating treat. I would put some toast on and get out coffee and creamer. I would place the toast on a saucer and sometimes several chocolate-covered biscuits as well. After three or four cups of coffee, I had major jitters. I would suddenly realize that I had been reading the same sentence over and over for at least ten minutes without taking in a single word.

During my long-night sugar and coffee vigils, I developed agitated stress patterns. Still awake at three a.m., but unable to continue studying, I would bite my nails and pull out my hair. I also started face-picking. It did not occur to me that chemical addiction might be the cause. I thought I was going insane.

When I started working as a waitress at an Italian bistro, I met the double espresso. I started to work at five a.m. I had two double shots of espresso then and by lunchtime I required two more. By the time I finished my shift, I felt totally drained.

It was just a matter of time before I turned to another stimulant: methamphetamine. There were late-night clubs where I could find it. Stressed from work, I would go there, pay about £20 for some powder, and then dance my brains out. I considered this my release from work; but it was the same cycle: exhaustion and overstimulation, which continued the all-night-studying pattern. The illegal drug use and all night partying just added to my problems.

I was only 21. I had gained weight, couldn't sleep, was constantly stressed, and had bad acne. My body was stiff. I was depressed and too anxious to leave the house.

I had lack of confidence. I doubted my mind's ability to take on new information. I could change my course load, my lifestyle, or my job, but I was taught to work as hard as I could so that I could have a good job. I was determined to be a success even if it meant sacrificing my health.

This isn't just a rant about how miserable life can be; there is a connection. Caffeine, sugar, and methamphetamine are all stimulants.

When I discovered this through online research, I realized that each of my addictions had contributed to the other. Caffeine, as a "gateway drug," had increased my dependence on other substances. It had been the first drug that I had ever tried, and the first to whack out my system so that I had become stimulant dependent. Caffeine had been leaving me in a constant state of exhausted overstimulation.

Caffeine and sugar are snuck into soft drinks and packaged foods. To detoxify myself from these stimulants, I drank water and ate nothing but pasta, rice, potatoes, bananas, zucchini, and spinach. I had nothing sweet; my only treat was a green vegetable and fruit juice. I did not have coffee or any other stimulant.

After about three months, I had completely lost all traces of stress and insomnia. Not only did I wake naturally before my alarm sounded, but I had so much energy that I did a yoga routine every day after breakfast. My skin cleared, I dropped weight, and my hair became shinier. I felt so much better about myself that I made friends, including my current boyfriend.

I still have to be vigilant about stimulants. When I had a job in a small, friendly office, whoever got up to make coffee would offer the others a cup. At first I would accept a cup and let it sit until it got cold. Then I revealed that I had caffeine problems. Without sounding officious or being haughty, I explained that my body reacts differently to caffeine; in fact, some of my co-workers had problems, too. Because of my honesty, I made new friends.

My policy of not drinking coffee was inexplicable to most people. "She doesn't drink coffee," my boss would say. I would just smile away my irritation, remaining firm in my conviction. Coffee is viewed as a substance with benefits, not dangers. It's one of those "harmless addictions." We write off the hours of stress for a few moments of pleasure, but then we wind up paying for it physically, even psychologically. Caffeine is not harmless if it causes health problems.

Now I listen to my body and take it easy when it comes to stress and workload. With the right diet and healthy alternatives to caffeinated or sugary drinks, I no longer crave stimulants. The aroma of coffee only reminds me how far I have come.

~ 15th Confession ~
My Vomiting Pill

I cannot recall the specific day when I first had coffee or tried an energy drink, but I will never forget the day I decided to quit.

My addiction to caffeine started when I went to college. On a typical day, I would chug four to five cups of coffee. Sometimes I would chase the coffee with a sugar-packed energy drink. If I didn't have time to go to the coffee shop before class, I would feel edgy for the rest of the day. I believed coffee made me accomplish more, but in actuality I was so jittery that I was probably less efficient. I became known for spilling my coffee in journalism class. Once, when I was hyped up on coffee, I spilled my java across the conference table during my professor's lecture. I felt embarrassed, but it was more than that. Coffee also changed my personality. I was impatient, short-tempered, and easily irritated.

My justification for drinking coffee kept me addicted. I worked two jobs to put myself through college, and I was always searching for additional energy. It was a delicate balance. If I consumed more or less than my usual coffee dose for a day, the result was a severe headache and fits of vomiting. Any noise or light would make my migraines symptoms worse. The only antidote: sleep in a dark, quiet room.

The first time I overdosed on coffee, I had to drive an hour and a half home from work in rush hour traffic, stopping to throw up along the way. For years I suffered from coffee-induced migraines. After the migraines set in, I would always vow to quit coffee, just like an alcoholic promises not to drink after a night of binge drinking. My breath, hair, and skin reeked of coffee. It felt as if it was seeping out of my pores. The problem was that I loved coffee. I drank it with friends and family members and could not imagine handling my workload without caffeine. It was socially acceptable and comforting, why should I quit? So I continued to suffer from migraines and kept on drinking coffee.

Then I finally had enough. It was summer, and I was living in Honolulu. I was assigned to interview a teenager who was attempting to be the youngest person to circumnavigate the globe. I had just hit the coffee shop to buy an extra-large black coffee. Holding the hot coffee in my hand, I was at the harbor waiting while a staff photographer corralled a speedboat, so we could get exclusive shots and an interview with the young sailor before he docked. I nearly slipped getting onto the boat, but I didn't drop my cup. We sped around the teenager's sailboat, snapping photographs and yelling questions at him. As we raced around the water, I juggled my recorder, notepad, and precious coffee.

The boat rocked back and forth, but I held onto my java. I genuinely believed that I could not be as productive without my coffee. After an hour on the water, I began to feel seasick, and the only comfort I had was a bitter—now cold—cup of coffee. I finished it before we docked, but I still felt my brain cells dragging. I decided to drain the last bit of java left in a coffeepot inside the harbor office. Even after two cups of black coffee, I felt my energy waning. Although I believed coffee gave me energy, the reality was that the caffeine crash depleted it more than anything else. When I got back to the office, I grabbed another cup of coffee at the liquor store downstairs. Before I took the last swig, my body was already shaky. I was doomed to pay a heavy price for my obsession.

Hours later, my head was spinning as I tried to write the article. I remember the young circumnavigator's words as he anchored his boat: "Football season is starting now. They are all running, and I can barely stand." He said this after a month of sailing from California to Hawaii. I, too, could barely stand, but all I had done was drink three very large cups of black coffee. I felt sick.

I was running back and forth from my desk to the toilet, vomiting uncontrollably. It was not seasickness. The severe migraine was an indication that I had drunk too much coffee. I felt so sick that I did not care what the women in the neighboring stalls thought as they heard me lose my breakfast and lunch. Nothing helped the nausea, and the fluorescent lights in the newsroom seemed to glare like high-beams on a pick-up truck.

I was feverishly trying to finish the story. Just as I was about to run to the ladies' room for another barf break, my editor tapped me on the shoulder to tell me my story would appear on the front page. My head dropped into my sweaty palms. Usually journalists love the recognition front-page coverage brings, but getting the lead story meant I would have to type another paragraph for the cover page. I could barely work, and I had only a few hours before I had to go to my second job. Shaking from the migraine, I phoned my other boss and asked for a sick day. He joked that I should never combine boat trips and cheap coffee. All I could say was, "I don't drink cheap coffee." After I finished the article, I drove home, stopping intermittently to vomit on the street.

At home I lay in the cold bathtub in pain as pellets of water fell on my body. I swore to quit drinking coffee. I was tired of being sick. I was tired of missing work because of migraines. I was fed up with explaining my condition to friends, co-workers, and family members.

The next morning I figured I would feel better, but I was wrong.

The withdrawal symptoms turned out to be worse than the migraines. I vomited for four days straight, and I had to postpone work and school while I recovered.

Coffee did not agree with my system, and I was determined to stop. I had almost lost a front-page story by being sick from a coffee overdose. I decided no more coffee for me. The only question was—how would I get energy? I upped my exercise routine and changed my diet. Surprisingly, I found that I had more energy without coffee! I also took supplements and vitamins daily. My belief that coffee gave me additional energy turned out to be completely false. After quitting, I felt healthier and more productive. Best of all, my migraines disappeared—at least temporarily. Then I developed a dependence on black tea.

I started drinking one to two cups of tea a day. Slowly, as my obligations increased, so did my tea intake. I never thought I would suffer from debilitating migraines again, but I was wrong.

One day before work, I drank about four to five cups of tea on an empty stomach. By the time I got to work, I had thrown up twice—once in a crowded McDonald's bathroom and later on the curb in front of work. Twenty minutes into work, I had to leave because I was running back and forth to the bathroom. Since the unisex bathroom was located near my co-worker's desk, I did not even have to explain. He heard me vomit up the Sprite I bought at the liquor store after I had vomited at the McDonald's.

I know my reaction and dependence on caffeine is not unusual, although it is extreme. Just in my circle of co-workers and friends, I know numerous people who drink coffee despite migraines. They are addicted, just like I was. We are overworked and sleep-deprived, looking for supplemental energy.

I still crave coffee. Whenever someone is brewing coffee, I stop to inhale the aroma. I sometimes cave in and drink a cup, but I always become sick afterward and have a migraine. Although I often cannot fight my cravings, I have eliminated caffeine from my daily routine. For me—the undergraduate who was inseparable from her coffee mug—that is a huge accomplishment. Quitting coffee and tea meant changing my life. For years I had been accustomed to toting around my coffee mug. I spent a lot of time and money on coffee and coffee accessories. I still have my collectable coffee mugs in my cupboard. I even had the perfect purse with a large outside pocket for my mug.

On the plus side, deciding to stop drinking tea and coffee meant white teeth, fresh breath, and extra pocket change. After I kicked my caffeine addiction, I would not have to whiten my teeth or carry around perfume to disguise the coffee odor.

Now I do not suffer from migraine headaches. I have more natural energy, and if I need an energy boost, I exercise, get some fresh air, and drink lots of water. My caffeine addiction was a terrible ordeal for me; I'm still thrilled that it's over.

~ 16th Confession ~
Stay Away from Caffeine!

Caffeine crept into my life like the slow drip of a percolating pot of Columbian dark.

I started drinking coffee in my freshman year of college. I was studying at Northern Illinois University in DeKalb, Illinois, the birthplace of barbed-wire. The setting would drive anybody to reach for something to kill the pain of cloudy days and cold nights.

DeKalb was in the middle of corn country, and the land was flat and low. The wind would come howling off the plains of Canada, through North Dakota and Minnesota, and into Northern Illinois. There was nothing to stop it. I'd be chilled to the bone by the time I walked from the dorm to the library.

To warm up, I always stopped at the library canteen. Hot cocoa was my choice. One evening when I went to the vending machine, the hot chocolate selection was empty. The only option was coffee. I deposited a quarter in the machine. Down dropped the cup and in poured the hot brew. I was on my way.

That first night, I felt the quick buzz from the caffeine. After that, coffee became my steady habit. I could rely on it to alter my mood, sharpen my focus, and get me through the arduous hours of studying.

Hot cocoa was now too juvenile for me. Coffee was an adult drink and I loved it.

The years passed. I transferred schools, graduated, got a job, and eventually married. I met my wife over a cup of coffee during my senior year of college. I first met her in the college bookstore. We took the conversation down the street to the corner cafe. High on caffeine, we spent the rest of the evening talking about literature, movies, and aspirations.

My wife wasn't the only person I met over coffee. I met many friends, too. A cup of coffee was also a good excuse to shut down for a while and relax. That's what would make it so difficult to stop drinking coffee. I had arranged my life around coffee. My schedule was dictated by coffee breaks.

I didn't know I had a problem with caffeine until a physical exam. I had experienced discomfort in my chest for some time, a dull pain that would come and go. Occasionally it felt like my heart skipped a beat. It was most prevalent and noticeable while I was at rest. I knew I should have these symptoms checked out, but I was young and invincible—what could be the problem?

What drew me to the doctor's office wasn't chest pain, but a hiking trip I planned to take with my wife. She persuaded me to make a visit to the doctor first to check my lower back, another nagging issue. The doctor reassured me that my back was fine. As the exam continued, he put the stethoscope against my chest. "Breathe in and hold it. Okay, you can let go. Again, breathe in and hold it. Let go," he said. He looked concerned.

"You know you have a murmur?" It was both a question and a statement.

"No, I didn't know. What does that mean?" I asked him. I was scared.

"I'll need you to have some tests to evaluate it," he said.

The problem seemed to be with the heart valve. It wasn't closing. "I'll setup an EKG, echo, and a stress test," the doctor said.

He couldn't tell the extent of my problem, but he knew it was serious. I was only 27. I'm too young for this, I thought.

It was a bright June morning when I went for the tests. The sun blasted through a window into the waiting room. Across from me sat an attractive middle-aged woman. I felt groggy, irritated, and nervous. I had been told not to have any caffeine before I went for the echocardiogram.

The woman must have sensed my anxiety. We were in the cardiac wing of the hospital, so we were both here for the same reason.

"Do you have to have an echo?" she asked. I nodded.

She explained that she had been living with mitral valve prolapse for nearly a decade.

"Is there anything I can do to stop the progression of the problem?" I asked.

"Stay away from caffeine," she said.

I told her how I loved that first cup of coffee in the morning, looked forward to my mid-morning brew, had an afternoon pick-me-up, and closed out my day with a cup after dinner.

She nodded her head in agreement and then let me know that all would have to change. "That's the way it was, but not the way it's going to be. The fluttering feeling will only get worse and coffee may exacerbate your problem," she said.

These were harsh words.

It's been ten years since I met that woman. When I go for my annual echocardiogram, I look for her. I haven't spotted her since, and I wonder what became of her. Did she have surgery? I did twice.

It wasn't until I underwent the second surgery that I finally weaned myself off caffeine. I'll occasionally have a cup in the morning, but my day isn't ruled by it anymore. The irritation I used to feel if I didn't get a cup was gone. My relationship with my wife has improved. I'm not as short-tempered as I used to be. I'm better off both physically and mentally. The heart murmur made me reevaluate my life, habits, and decisions. It was the one of the best and worst things to happen to me.

~ 17th Confession ~
Divine Intervention

I grew up in a family of coffee lovers in the buzzing city of Mumbai. The rule at home, however, was that children should not be permitted to drink beverages like tea and coffee until they entered their teens. So, even though the coffee aroma always tempted me as a child, it was only on the evening of my thirteenth birthday that I first tasted it. Little did I realize the influence this first mug of coffee and the effect it would have on my life.

Coffee soon became a part of my daily routine. I woke up to a steaming mug of coffee in the morning and topped it off with more cups during the day. I loved coffee and never tired of it. It became my staple and my midmorning fuel—the taste of other drinks paled by comparison. My coffee intake was a minimum of four large mugs and a maximum of ten on days when I was staying up late preparing for college exams.

When I married, I moved in with my husband's family—also big coffee enthusiasts. Every other hour, there would be rounds of coffee prepared for everyone. If we had any visitors, we would serve them coffee as well, and the entire family would join in, having yet another cup for the day.

Through all those years, I did not realize what coffee was doing to my sleep pattern. As I was edging toward my mid-twenties, I began staying up later more than usual. This happened

97

over a period of years. I could not easily slip off to sleep and would stay up almost half the night tossing and turning.

At first, I attributed these insomniac patterns to the changes in my environment—a new home, new people around me—and I thought perhaps I was inwardly struggling to settle down. However, things did not get any better, even after two years of marriage. I could not fall asleep until late at night and struggled to wake up on time every morning.

Like most married women, I was eager to start a family. My husband and my in-laws were equally keen. We had not used any contraceptives for the first two years of our marriage, yet I had not conceived. Oddly, I did not find this unusual.

Then began the months and months of trying to conceive. I had already celebrated my twenty-eighth birthday, and the pressure was mounting from my family and in-laws. Back home in India, neighbors took as much of an interest in my life as did my family. Questions were asked; eyebrows were raised: Isn't she almost 30? Are they still not trying for a baby?

For nearly two years, we tried to have a child—keeping a chart, understanding the fertile time of the month, and so forth. Our efforts were in vain. By then, my self-esteem had hit an all-time low. Why was I being singled out by God? When would the neighbors stop talking? This entire thought process stressed me out even more and compounded my insomniac tendencies.

Finally, heeding advice from my family and friends, my husband and I decided to consult a doctor who specialized in fertility treatments. He ran a series of tests on both of us. All results were normal. My husband's sperm count was fine, and my hormone levels were perfect. The doctor said, "Stress can cause delays in conceiving. So just relax. Stop thinking about it. There is nothing wrong with either of you. Just keep trying."

Just keep trying? Wasn't that exactly what I had been doing for the last three years? This abnormality—as I began calling it —was driving me nuts. I had frequent spells of weepiness. My relationship with my husband began deteriorating as I picked frequent quarrels with him for the smallest reasons. I began getting on his nerves with my constant mood swings, which only got worse with my inability to sleep. I used to lie awake in bed until the wee hours while he slept peacefully, which exasperated me even more.

One day I bumped into an old college mate who had begun practicing naturopathy. This friend began explaining what she did, how she started believing in natural cures for common ailments after a life-altering incident in her life. We chatted for a long time, sitting in a restaurant, and during our conversation, she learned about my inability to conceive.

Providence, I would call it. My meeting her at that opportune time was divine intervention. Within ten minutes of telling her about my plight—about the medical tests, my cycles, and my diet patterns—she said one word: caffeine.

She began mulling over my problem, asking seemingly irrelevant questions about my diet. Finally, she announced, "It's the coffee that is the culprit. Stop or at least reduce your consumption of coffee. Here's my number. Call me anytime you want."

To me, this sounded totally absurd. I was aware that coffee contained caffeine, but I did not look at it as a drug that could be harmful. All the adults in my family and my in-laws had been drinking coffee for years. Everyone was still alive with no major health concerns, and none of the married women had any difficulty conceiving—therefore, it did not make sense. Could she have a point? I wasn't sure, but I kept thinking about her words all through my journey home that evening.

I resolved to give her theories a shot. I had nothing to lose. I did not try to give up coffee completely. I knew I didn't have it in me to give up a habit that had been with me for over 15 years. My body demanded coffee every morning. I tried to reduce the amount in each cup, but after an hour or so, I would take another half cup to appease my craving. This went on day after day. After about a week, I realized that I had actually cut down a cup or two. Hurray!

All through this ordeal, I had only my naturopath friend to depend on for moral support. My husband's family did not notice that I was trying to reduce my consumption of caffeine. I did not want them to scoff at me. Nor did I confide in my husband.

I became aware that if I could reduce a cup or two in one week's time, I had the strength to reduce my consumption of coffee even more. I will not deny that I had weak moments when I wanted to give in to the temptation of having a cup during the day. Like cigarette smoking, it is a mental trick to have coffee as a quick fix to any problem. After drinking that cup, I could fool myself into believing that the caffeine did me some good, but nothing would be further from the truth.

Week after week, I steadfastly continued. In eight weeks, I had reduced my coffee intake to just two cups in the morning. It had been one of the most difficult times of my life. Giving up the afternoon cup was the hardest as I believed that it perked me up and kept me going for the rest of the day. When I eventually gave up that afternoon cup, it helped to cure my insomnia. I was thrilled. It had been coffee all along!

Because I began sleeping better, my mood improved, and I was less irritable with my husband. The neighbors' talk did not bother me anymore. I was able to smile it off, inwardly thinking that I might just surprise you all in six months. Just you wait and watch. My ability to sleep better greatly contributed to my positive frame of mind during the day, which in turn contributed to a healthy dose of lovemaking at night. I realize now how important sleep is to our physical and mental well-being.

My menstrual cycles, meanwhile, continued to be as regular as ever. I continued to talk to my naturopath friend off and on. We seemed to be in constant telephone contact ever since the fateful day that we met.

Then it happened—I missed a cycle! I was jubilant, but wanted to wait a few more days before I went in for a test. Every morning I would wake up wondering if this could really be happening. Two weeks later, my doctor confirmed that I was pregnant!

I will admit that I had been a skeptic. I would have attributed all of this to mere coincidence or the result of reduced stress. Maybe solving the insomnia problem was a part of the solution, but more than anything, I believe caffeine had caused my infertility.

I will not lie and say I have entirely given up coffee. I still enjoy my one and only morning cup, but I can live without it. On the days that I don't get coffee, I don't break into a sweats or get headaches like I used to.

Now, thanks to the Internet and information-rich Web sites, I have found enough evidence against caffeine: its links to insomnia, infertility, the mind's dependence on caffeine, and so much more.

When I look back on my ordeal of curing infertility by reducing caffeine, I marvel at the simplicity of it all. Sometimes, the best things in life are surprisingly simple. If only we knew how to be aware of them.

~ 18th Confession ~
Moment of Clarity

Stimulants—legal or illegal? Pick your poison. Caffeine was my drug of choice and the only way to make it through the day.

At age seven I began having difficulty waking up for school, so my mother would give me Coca-Col with my breakfast. Then she replaced my lunchtime juice with Coke. Soon I had soda with every meal. It took a lot more than one can to get the buzz, but I was allowed as much as I wanted.

My caffeine intake was increasing in an attempt to combat sleepiness. It was not normal that a child was always sleepy and unable to function without high doses of caffeine My sleepiness indicated some kind of disorder, but masking it with caffeine had serious consequences. It turned out that I had Hodgkin's disease (lymphoma). By the time it was discovered, no one was sure how long I'd had it. During chemotherapy I used Coca-Cola to keep going and to hold nausea at bay, unaware that drinking it was probably doing more harm than good. Despite lack of knowledge about what was healthy, I battled cancer and won.

When I got well, I began playing tennis and caffeine played a role in that part of my life as well. Instead of water, I drank soda during competition. Many athletes who appeared in TV commercials were portrayed as being able to reach their achievements because they drank Coke or Pepsi. It seems ridiculous when I look at this as an adult. As a teen, it was not much of a stretch to believe that Coca-Cola would make me superhuman and that the crash was not because of the caffeine but a lack of it. So I drank soda before, during, and after matches. I did not realize that I might have played better without caffeine.

My chronic sleepiness continued, so I kept using caffeine to boost my energy. In college I discovered NoDoz, Vivarin, and their generic counterparts. I could get the jolt I needed without soda. I soon lost the taste for soda, which was an indication that I was using it only for the caffeine—it was a chemical dependence. Taking a pill was easier than downing ounces of carbonated liquid. I no longer had to suffer from the tooth decay or the bloating in my stomach. I thought I had died and gone to heaven. I did not realize that the pills would place me in purgatory.

It was as hard to wake up as it had always been, so I would set an alarm one hour before the time I needed to be awake and put a bottle of water and caffeine pills next to my bed. When the alarm rang, I swallowed a pill and fell back asleep for an hour. During this hour, one or two things would happen: My heart would begin racing and I would wake up or I would have an urgency to urinate or have a bowel movement. As a result, I would jump out of the bed. But over time, one pill would not work, so I would take two. Then two stopped working, and I took four. I would take another pill before class and then crash and take two more in the afternoon.

I realized this was not a great way to live, so during semester breaks I would stop using pills, sleep as much as I wanted, and drink gallons of water. After the break, I would begin caffeine intake again. This continued throughout college. My life was a constant battle to stay awake and function, so I could not quit caffeine completely.

After college I went to work, and caffeine continued its control over me. I struggled to maintain a normal routine. I was always tired, so I supplemented the caffeine pills with coffee. My caffeine intake was raised to new heights. This did bother me, but the sleepiness bothered me more. I could have a cup of coffee right before bed and fall asleep, no problem. I would sleep a lot and still feel tired. I had to urinate constantly, sometimes my kidneys ached, and I was dehydrated. Caffeine also made me obnoxious. I was juiced up and annoying at times. It hurt my relationship with my friends and family. My life was hell, but I was addicted to something that is not considered a big deal. That is how I tried to justify it.

One day I was invited to participate in a cancer research study at the hospital where I had been treated as a youth. I decided to go. The tests showed that my sleepiness, missed for almost 20 years by doctors, despite my complaints that I am really lethargic, sluggish, and exhausted all the time, was a result of hormones that were out of whack. I had been compensating with caffeine and masking a serious health problem.

What to do was clear. I would get the treatment I needed and I would change my lifestyle. No more caffeine. Only water. No more fast food. I would exercise: weight training, stretching, cardio—everything. It is the only way to be healthy.

~ 19th Confession ~
Wake Up and Smell the Coffee

I grew up in a house where a fresh pot of coffee was always brewing. The smell of the roasted beans permeated the house and created a warm, welcoming environment. When we had company, everyone accepted a cup. It was part of offering hospitality. My mother and father would sit together every morning and share conversation over coffee. It seemed to bring them together before my father went to work.

I started drinking coffee when I was eight. I would steal a sip or two from my parents' cups when they weren't looking. I preferred my father's sweetened creamy coffee to my mother's black, unsweetened drink. Eventually, my parents bought me my own coffee cup, and I was invited to sit with them in the mornings and enjoy this wonderful brew. They didn't see any harm in it, and it was nice to sit together and share conversation or just enjoy the morning's peacefulness.

During my college years, I used coffee, caffeine gum, and soda to stay up late and study. At that time, coffeehouses and drive-thru coffee huts were becoming popular. Espresso, cappuccino, café latte—I acquired a taste for stronger, higher quality brews with each drink I tried. I loved smelling the coffee beans while they were being ground and brewed. I enjoyed watching the baristas, carefully creating designs in the froth. I envied their skill and learned about brewing by talking with them. I savored the first brisk sip of coffee and felt warmed by my drink.

I began visiting coffee hangouts every day, sometimes more than once a day. The baristas knew exactly how I liked my drinks: strong, light, and sweet. If they saw me coming, they would start on my drink.

I suffered a few nights when I couldn't sleep, but I loved how alert I became with each cup. I could be in a rotten mood and turn it around in less than five minutes with one cup of coffee. I was becoming an addict—in a harmless way, or so I thought.

After I finished college, I worked for a large publishing company. It was a fulfilling job, and when the company's CEO installed a coffee bar in the lobby of our building that only made the job sweeter. My co-workers and I rotated the job of coffee-gofer every morning, and I sneaked down for my own cup in the afternoon, sometimes followed by a handful of chocolate-covered coffee beans.

During one of my visits to the coffeehouse, I met Jake. Before I knew it, we were together all the time. Unbeknownst to me, he had his own addictions—street drugs and alcohol. We were married, and then his problem with drugs came out. He tried to whitewash it as purely recreational use, but he used marijuana, heroin, and alcohol daily. I had never experimented with drugs or alcohol, so I didn't understand his dependence, and I pressured him to get over it. I thought he could kick the habit, but when he tried, he was irritable and despondent. He said he felt like a failure when he fell short of my expectations, so I stopped urging him to quit. Often, he chided me for all the coffee I drank and challenged me to stop drinking it. I told him I would quit if he would kick his habits, so we tried together. It was the most miserable week of my life. I had terrible headaches. I couldn't deal with Jake and he couldn't deal with me. We both quickly fell off the wagon.

Jake started to bait me into arguments and criticize me over petty things, not just the amount of coffee I drank, but what I ate and how I dressed. He would count the money I spent on coffee, although we didn't talk about the money he poured into his addiction. I started to hide my bankcard receipts from the coffee shops or pay with cash, and I evaded any conversation about how I spent my money.

About a year into our marriage, after much soul-searching, I asked for a divorce. It was bad timing. I found out that I was pregnant. We agreed to work on our problems, stay together, and have the baby. We had an unspoken agreement to leave each other alone about our addictions.

My pregnancy was difficult, and I was deflated when I had to quit my job. I was even more upset when the doctor told me to stay away from caffeine completely, including coffee. But coffee seemed to temper my morning sickness and felt comforting. The doctor reluctantly allowed me one 6-ounce cup, but warned me about the potential problems if I drank more. I cut back to one 20-ounce cup per day.

After my daughter was born, I developed postpartum depression. I was alert—too alert—and hypersensitive. I became agoraphobic and was afraid to venture outside even to the mailbox. I cut off everyone except my husband and baby daughter. I ignored calls from my old boss to come back to work. Jake discouraged me from going back, reminding me how it would shortchange our child if I put her into daycare. I felt guilty, isolated, and helpless.

I had inherited my mother's habit of always keeping coffee brewing while I was home. Having that pot helped me stay awake. I felt tired all the time, and caffeine helped perk me up.

Besides, it was comforting, reminding me of old times and my mother and father sharing conversation and coffee. However, there was a distinct difference between the diner-style coffee that my mother made and the dark-roasted espresso blend that I brewed. As I drank my first cup in the morning, I thought back to the closeness my parents had and realized how different my marriage felt.

By the time Jake came home from work, I would be so high-strung from all the coffee that I was bouncing off the walls while he was tired. He shut me out, ignoring me for the entire evening. Most weekends, he left me alone with our daughter and went out with co-workers or to find drugs.

To bring in extra income, I stayed up nights working on freelance projects, brewing a new pot of coffee after my family went to bed. I was depriving myself of sleep at night and a social life during the day.

One day I received e-mail from an old college friend. She wanted to get together and catch up on old times. I felt anxious about meeting someone whose life was probably much more successful than mine. I felt like a mess and I looked like one. I gathered up my courage and met her at a coffee shop. After meeting with her a few times, I started to feel better about venturing out. Jake did not like that I left our daughter with a babysitter, but I needed to get out of the house, so I went against his wishes. My friend could see how reclusive I had become and suggested I see a counselor. At first I felt criticized, but after she pointed out how dysfunctional my life had become, seeing a counselor seemed like a good idea. With her help and prodding, and without my husband's knowledge, I found a counselor. After breaking three appointments, I finally forced myself to go.

The counselor told me that I needed to "clean house" and get my life in balance. The first thing she said was to give up my addiction to caffeine, to start exercising everyday. She told me to avoid replacing coffee with some other form of caffeine. I was scared. She was telling me to give away my crutch. I remembered that week of hell when I had tried to quit previously, but I followed her instructions.

By exercising and drinking water, I avoided the worst of the withdrawal symptoms. Once I stopped depending on caffeine, I began sleeping normally and eating more healthfully. I broke the habit of putting a pot on in the morning and cut back on the amount of work I tackled during the evening. Within two weeks of this new routine, I knew what I needed to do. I put my daughter into daycare and found a job.

Leaving behind my addiction to caffeine not only made me feel healthier, but it also gave me the confidence to leave my marriage. Very little happiness came from it; I was consumed by Jake's needs and expectations, and I had been clinging to the comforts of my childhood.

Now when I walk by a coffee stand, the aroma brings back memories, both good and bad. Sometimes I feel the urge to buy a cup. Then I remember my progress away from that chemical crutch, and I keep walking.

~ 20th Confession ~
Caffeine Nightmare

I never did drugs, but in college I became addicted to the unlikeliest of drugs, caffeine.

During my sophomore year, I was taking 15 credits while working part-time and writing for the school newspaper. My body and mind could not keep up. I was falling asleep in class and on the job. I began looking for ways to increase my energy. A floor-mate suggested coffee. I hated coffee, but I thought I would try it. I ordered a large cup of black coffee from the campus cafeteria while studying for a test. It was very bitter and I had trouble finishing it. By the end of the hour, I understood why people flocked to caffeine. I felt re-energized and was easily able to finish studying. That began an addiction that has not ended to this day.

I would buy three cups of black coffee and stay up as long as I needed. I had enough energy to study and work both jobs. I thought this is how Superman must feel, finding a way to attain limitless energy. Caffeine seemed to be too good to be true, and I would find out that it was.

After drinking three cups of black coffee a day for a year, my body started to crave even more caffeine. I started to buy Jolt soda, which was advertised as having twice the strength as coffee. Buying three cups of coffee and a six-pack of Jolt a day started crippling my finances. Then I added energy drinks.

Even though I was working two jobs, my income was not enough to buy enough caffeine to keep me alert. I started borrowing money from my parents and friends to make ends meet, but I was never able to catch up to my newfound debt.

Physically, things became just as tough. I got headaches when I did not get enough caffeine. I also felt sluggish, nervous, and grumpy. My concentration and focus waned, and my schoolwork and job production plummeted. I had mood swings. I would be happy and pleasant, but in an instant I would get angry and impatient. My girlfriend fought with me because of this and demanded that I stop drinking coffee and soda, but that infuriated me even more. The time we spent together erupted into heated arguments. We eventually broke up. I still have regrets, though I have not heard from her for many years.

Additionally, I would get into arguments with my parents. Before my addiction, we had a close and loving relationship. But they started questioning my constant requests for money. I would shout at them and hang up on them. I could not control myself.

Caffeine was already having a devastating effect, but things would get even worse. In high school, I was diagnosed with high blood pressure and a heart murmur. For years after the diagnosis, I have never had any problems. However, my high caffeine intake made my heart and blood pressure race, putting me in constant danger of a heart attack, but I could not quit.

Near the end of my junior year, I had two major exams. I decided I would pull two all-nighters of studying. At five p.m. I drank five cups of black coffee and six cans of Jolt. Then I had five energy drinks and took three pills of Vivarin, a caffeine drug. The commercials advertised that it was just as safe as coffee. I would soon find out the commercials were wrong.

By nine p.m. I started getting heart palpitations, felt nauseous, broke out in a cold sweats, and became very jittery. I wanted to overcome these physical disorders using mental strength, but that was futile. I felt dizzy and thought I would collapse right in the study room. I continued to feel worse and worse.

Two hours later, I started experiencing hallucinogenic images. The words from my textbook came off the pages and danced in front of me. I started hearing voices. They got louder and louder, swearing at me and mocking me. I put my hands over my ears, but the sounds would not stop. I was now in full panic mode and ran downstairs to my dorm room. As I entered the room, my poster of Jimmy Hendrix lunged at me. The image of Hendrix was trying to grab me. I jumped away from his hand and then dove under the covers of my bed. I prayed for the horror to stop, but the prayers had no effect on my agony. I felt crawling bugs underneath my skin. I scratched feverishly to stop the invaders, cutting myself with my scratches. I screamed for help, but no one came to my aid. Sweat poured down, my heart raced, and I thought the end was coming soon. Scared and in agony, I collapsed in my bed.

I woke up two days later. Bedridden for three days, I was dehydrated and exhausted as if I had run a marathon. I ended up missing both my exams. A doctor said the caffeine overdose put my already weak heart at risk and I was fortunate that I survived.

After I almost met my Creator, I should quit, but I have not. I only learned to be careful with caffeine. I drink at least three cups of coffee a day, continue to drink energy drinks, but I do not take caffeine pills. Although I am able to control my caffeine intake, I have not been able to end it. My body demands it and I cannot resist. You can get addicted to caffeine just like to any other drug; and just like any other drug, it can be dangerous.

~ 21st Confession ~
My Struggle

My name is Sarah, and I am an addict. I grew up in a dysfunctional alcoholic family... What you are told in therapy and in underage drinking prevention programs is that alcohol is a "gateway drug." However, my "gateway drug" was caffeine. I was addicted to caffeine before I knew that it was an addictive substance, but I didn't realize it until I tried to quit.

I was working at a fast food restaurant and going to school. When I started to work, I was handed a uniform and a 32-ounce cup, which I could fill with as much soda as I wanted. Awesome! My parents never provided that much soda, so I thought it was great.

Not long after I started working, I began experiencing heart palpitations. I didn't realize it was related to the caffeine in the soda. I was consuming about a gallon of Dr. Pepper a day. Eventually, I got so sick of the taste that I quit drinking it cold turkey.

A few days after my sudden break from caffeine, I got the worst migraines I'd ever had. I felt sick, continually throwing up, and spent days lying in the dark with a cold cloth on my head. After three weeks of pain, I went to the doctor. I told him I'd quit drinking soda about three weeks prior. He smiled and said, "I'll be right back." I figured he would write a prescription for some great migraine medication. Instead, he walked into the room with a can of Dr. Pepper and said, "Take two of these and call me in the morning." He explained that most people have to taper off caffeine to avoid the horrendous headaches that I was experiencing. He told me to drink one soda a day, then every other day, and keep lowering my caffeine intake. I swore I would never become a caffeine addict again.

A few years later, I was pregnant with my first child. To combat my morning sickness, which had gotten so bad that I required intravenous hydration and was on medication to keep me from throwing up, I started to drink Pepsi. It was the beginning of a caffeine addiction that would imprison me for the next 11 years.

I started to drink 32 ounces of Coke or Pepsi every day. This doubled to 64, then 96 ounces. I felt miserable. I couldn't get rid of the baby weight, and my breasts hurt. I had constant pain and all sorts of nodules in my breasts. I was diagnosed with fibrocystic breast disease. The pain grew worse, and I began having headaches again. One doctor or another told me to stop drinking soda, and I would try, but I couldn't. I was hooked and hated myself for returning to that point. I tried tapering off, but any time I felt stress I relapsed.

Some people told me that I was making mountains out of molehills because it was just soda. Why should I complain about an addiction to caffeine when I'd already quit smoking and was beating alcoholism? I began attending an addiction recovery program through my church, which perplexed some of my friends even more.

I knew I was dumping empty calories into my body, but every time I stopped drinking soda, the withdrawal symptoms were so horrible that I gave up. I'd always been sensitive to medications, never realizing the full effect of the non-prescribed drug that I was ingesting daily. I began to have panic attacks. Rosacea appeared on my face. I was plagued with insomnia and frequent urinary tract infections. My stomach began to revolt, causing cramps and diarrhea. My parents told me stories about people they knew who had gotten sick and it had been linked to sodas with artificial sweeteners. I figured that I didn't need to worry because I was drinking regular full-sugar soda, not the diet versions containing artificial sweeteners.

As my life was slowly crashing, I was constantly in a state of chaos: I always felt stressed, I yelled at my kids a lot, and I hated myself. I wasn't comfortable in my own skin. I started seeing a therapist, but I never brought up my caffeine addiction because I didn't want to be judged as a crazy person, though I probably was. I was so stressed out, unhappy, and physically ill that I truly believed I had gone crazy. So did some of the people who were close to me. They didn't understand the addiction, and I hardly understood it myself. Every couple of months, I tried to taper off. Then a stressful event would happen that I would use as an excuse to give up. There was one reason after another that I used to justify why I couldn't quit. I'd been thinking about quitting, I desperately wanted to quit, but I couldn't do it.

About a year ago, I really was going to quit. I found a lump in my breast and was going to undergo a surgical biopsy. Two days before I had surgery, my children flooded our bathroom and caused damage to our brand new home. This was my reason to stay hooked, even though I'd tapered off enough to be down to a 12-ounce can of Coke per day and already bought 6-ounce cans. There was a mixture of relief and self-loathing at the same time. I thought I would quit later, after I got the mess cleaned up. Then it was "as soon as the holidays are over." Then, "let me get through Great-Grandma's funeral."

I finally came to understand one critical point: The stress was not going to stop, but I had to. Armed with Excedrin and a resolve to finally break my addiction, I gave myself a day to gear up and quit cold turkey. I was very short-tempered and sometimes downright mean. Every time I started to get a headache, I took an Excedrin. I was slowly able to increase the time between doses, until one day I realized that three days had passed since my last dose. But for almost three weeks not a single day went by that I didn't crave a Coke. I was in the habit of buying a Coke from McDonald's every morning. They have the best mix, and it turned out to be a very difficult habit to break. On the twentieth day, my husband brought a Coke home from McDonald's.

Quick as a fox, I grabbed it, but he was faster. He took it away before I could even close my lips around the straw. I was furious. I screamed at him, told him that I hated him, and slammed the door. I felt desperate and nearly began to cry. Then, my ten-year-old son came up and told me he hoped I got over my caffeine addiction soon. Almost instantly, I began to feel better. My desire for Coke was gone. God had answered my prayers. The next morning came, and I still didn't crave one. The next morning, I still was okay. I am really thankful my husband took that Coke from me.

It's been almost ten weeks since I've had a Coke. Although I don't have the constant urge for caffeine and I am no longer counting hour by hour, it is still hard. The first time I ate at McDonald's after I quit I felt like a former alcoholic in a bar. A couple of weeks ago, my husband was out of town and I began to think that quitting was a mistake. Not having my husband around to hold me accountable, I knew I could buy a Coke and no one would ever know, but I also knew that if I had one Coke, I wouldn't be able to stop.

Quitting has definitely been worth it. I no longer get headaches and have more energy than I've had in a long time. My mood is better, my breasts don't hurt, and I no longer feel like a prisoner in my own body. I am not out of the woods, but I see the meadow, and it's gorgeous.

~ 22nd Confession ~
Caffeine+NASCAR=Speed

When I was 12, I went into my dad's race car garage and into his private office. Rummaging through his desk, I found a large zip-lock bag filled with hundreds of black and yellow capsules. Dad was a NASCAR driver, and a fan had given him a little more speed. These highly concentrated caffeine capsules were known as Black Beauties.

I filled my pocket, knowing my dad would never miss a few. I will never forget the next few days, feeling as if my scalp was crawling all over my head. This was my introduction to caffeine, and it made me feel unstoppable. Black Beauties and Yellow Jackets were just the beginning. As over-the-counter pills like 357 Magnums came on the scene, I was hooked.

Growing up in a NASCAR racing shop meant that I learned everything about car building and ultimately become a racing expert. By the time I was 30, the biggest teams and the best drivers were seeking me out. Running a race team is constant pressure with tight schedules, requiring the crew chief to be on site from early morning until late at night. For me, that required a steady dose of caffeine.

I started my day with a pill, filled in the middle with coffee, and then had soda followed by another couple of pills in the evening. It is ironic that I felt I was being responsible for not taking this apparently harmless drug to the next level: cocaine, crack, and meth. Then the bill came due.

I started to wake up in the mornings with nosebleeds. I could not figure out why until I decided to lay off caffeine for a day or so. This caused the nosebleeds to stop, but produced massive headaches. Any day that was not caffeine-assisted consisted of mood swings, feelings of frustration, and an energy level next to nothing. I decided that since the nosebleeds were in the morning, a few NoDoz or 357 Magnum pills in the afternoon would be okay.

I was naive. A dose taken early evening meant I would not get to sleep until after midnight, and that sleep was no longer sound. I could no longer awaken at my usual time and arrived at work incredibly late and with the worst disposition. Mechanics and engineers I had personally recruited spent hours without direction. Soon they started to complain and eventually quit.

I blamed all this on the high-powered caffeine pills. I was smart enough to see that anything in such high concentration could not be good for my body, no matter how good it made me feel, but this realization did not make me stop. Taking the same amount of caffeine at age 30 produced very different effects than at 18. My scalp no longer crawled, but my heart raced at an incredible rate, and I yawned and sweated at all hours of the day, never knowing when I would crash. My concentration shrank to nothing, leaving tasks incomplete and forgotten in the business where loose bolts could equal death to a driver or crew member.

I tried to cut out caffeine several times, always with the same failed result. My wife would buy caffeine-free drinks in an effort to do her part, but my body (or mind) rejected them as unpalatable. I could not stay awake during the day and could not sleep at night. Nosebleeds were constant and the mood roller coaster was never faster. I was so wound up that I could not relax on my days off, or even on vacation. My body shook. I was in a state of panic, feeling that this time was going to be wasted if I did not do some sort of productive work. I was the only person sitting on the beach working on my computer, and I did not see anything unusual with that.

My life had become a slave to the drug that no one warns you about. Moreover, companies pushing caffeine-laden soda, energy drinks, and coffee, even straight-up caffeine supplements, support and sponsor auto racing. One person on each team even has the specific job of making sure that cold caffeine is within reach of the crew at the track.

There is no way you are going to turn it down when you are working in 90-degree heat and your adrenaline is at 100 percent.

Then our race team hired a pit-crew coach. His job was to choreograph the pit stop moves, implement a workout schedule, and make sure that every member of the crew maintained a proper nutritional regimen. He explained a lot about caffeine that I had never known and the difference between stopping cold turkey and successfully reining in the beast.

His advice was to use lunchtime as a cut off point for all caffeine. The only fluid after one p.m. was water—no juice and no caffeine. He had no patience for the pills, calling my behavior very irresponsible. The pills had to go. In the morning, soda or coffee had to be kept to a minimum. I followed this advice, but it came too late to save my marriage.

As a father of two small kids, the only time I had to spend with my family was after my workday. Being a good father and husband meant being available for baths, bedtime stories, and intelligent late-night conversation. Caffeine robbed me of all that. I would fall asleep after reading just one page of a kid's book or during the most pivotal point of a conversation, leaving me looking and feeling like an uncaring ass. Work and sleep became the only two things in my life, and my wife divorced me.

Anyone who dismisses caffeine as less harmful or addictive as other drugs or alcohol is either stupid or an addict himself. I have now spent eight years off caffeine pills and about five years off caffeine-laden drinks, thanks to the nutritionist's advice. It has not been a cakewalk.

One day, I found a bottle of highly concentrated caffeine pills in the toolbox of a co-worker and immediately fell off the wagon. I found an excuse to borrow tools or whatever it took to take every pill, two at a time, day after day. The co-worker never said a word. I still wonder what his thoughts were and whether this is the reason that we do not work together anymore.

Day after day, I consumed cans of soda one after another. My brain blocked the memory that I just had a can and I would wind up opening another one. Then the same old symptoms such as shakes, feelings of panic, and nosebleeds came back.

I think it is sad that caffeine addicts don't have help such as Alcoholics Anonymous or Narcotics Anonymous. Like cocaine or alcohol, this drug can come back hard and fast. It only takes a cup of coffee to lead to a cold soda, and then I am off to the races.

The only remedy for me was to gradually remove caffeine and then remain diligent in keeping it out. Ginger ale has become a good friend. It tricks me into feeling as if I am consuming the bad stuff. If I avoid caffeine for a week or two, the headaches subside and I can get through my days smoothly and maintain consistent energy. A proper diet of vegetables, fish, chicken, and fresh fruit helps immensely, along with lots of water and a good exercise plan. Exercise is the "drug" that really works for you and your marriage.

The man who had given my dad the big bag of caffeine capsules told him that even though he was a fast driver, this stuff would make him go even faster. My dad accepted the gift, but never touched these pills. The Black Beauties stayed in the drawer until I found them. Dad never said a word about where they went or who had taken them. I wish he had punished me for swiping these pills or, better yet, thrown the entire lot into the garbage.

~ 23rd Confession ~
Drug Society

We live in the "Starbucks Age." The ultimate corporate enabler is located on every street corner, like a local drug dealer in a rough neighborhood. Everyone seems to be marching to the beat of caffeine: from home to work, during lunch, and during coffee breaks. For me, drinking at least three cups a day once seemed unavoidable, and soon went from being a convenient luxury to a daily necessity.

Starbucks symbolizes American affluence as much as it does our cultural addiction. The Declaration of Dependence on Caffeine (based on the Declaration of Independence as we know it) might read as follows: "We, the consumers, caffeine addicts of the United States of America, do solemnly swear to drink an excess of coffee every day."

When did we become so addicted to caffeine and why do only few people recognize this as a serious problem? Is it because smoking has always taken precedent? If so, now that those anti-smoking ads from the 1990s have done a number on the tobacco industry, maybe the caffeine industry should be the next target?

First, we should ask ourselves: Who is to blame for the widespread caffeine addiction? Is it Starbucks' fault or is it our own? Of course, Starbucks feeds off its increasingly addicted consumer base, but why are we so susceptible to addiction? Does our workaholic nature lead to our caffeine addictions or is it the other way around?

In America life moves faster. So must we, I used to think. We should always be working harder, staying focused longer—hour after hour, day after day. For a few bucks a cup, it never seemed wrong to get some help with keeping up this pace. How can we maintain the work ethic and discipline that we Americans pride ourselves on without ingesting heavy doses of caffeine? We have become accustomed to and reliant upon caffeine. Of course, Starbucks—the representative universal drug supplier—is always there for us, ready to provide another rush of caffeine.

The reason I preface my story with this diatribe is that it stems from America's enabler of caffeine addicts—Starbucks. Before my first year as a law student, I had never tasted coffee. As a kid, I had heard that coffee stunted growth, making me stay away from it as a teenager. I liked the smell of it, but coffee was for old fogies.

I began to feel the pressure during my first week of law school. Other students were constantly taking coffee breaks between class and while studying. There was a Starbucks inside the law school building, and another one right across the street. Sitting in the library, I would see every student, head buried in thick law books, with an oversized cup of coffee. I ordered my first cup just to fit in with the crowd. By the time I finished law school, I was drinking six, seven, sometimes more, large mugs a day. I inhaled the aroma of the freshly brewed roast and, since then, have not looked back—until this year.

I cannot think of a single day when I have not had a cup of coffee. Over the years, I have built up a tremendous tolerance to caffeine. One reason I drink so much coffee is the people around me do. My girlfriend Mary drinks coffee. Everyone in her family drinks coffee. Just being around her has increased the amount of coffee I consume. Coffee drinking is not only addictive, but it can also be contagious. When someone you're with drinks coffee, it's hard to refuse a cup.

Dunkin' Donuts' a recent TV ad proudly announces, "America runs on Dunkin.'" The ad suggests that coffee is an essential fuel, thereby turning an addiction into a vital necessity. Great advertising, indeed! Often, the goal of advertising is to make people want something they do not need or—even worse—need something that they don't want.

What better a product to play on that than coffee! Caffeine is a cash cow. It didn't take a marketing genius to realize how effectively a company can use the addictive quality of caffeine to boost sales by addicting consumers, which is exactly how corporate advertisers like Starbucks and Dunkin' Donuts work on a mass scale.

Mary and I decided to kick our addictions after we recognized our daily reliance on the coffee fuel. Initially, we switched to tea, but that lasted hardly three days. It turned out that we had to drink several cups of tea to get nearly the same feeling that we got from a cup of coffee, not to mention the inconvenient number of bathroom trips that accompany all that liquid. Drinking tea did not help decrease caffeine dependence. Our mental and physical reliance on this drug remained. We continued to "run" on caffeine.

Mary consulted a nutritionist/health nut friend. She didn't advice going cold turkey. Instead, she suggested we gradually consume less caffeine until we stopped entirely. We devised a regimen of decreasing caffeine intake. We would decrease the number of cups per day and slowly decrease the amount of caffeine in each cup.

At first, we drank our usual morning cup of coffee using 25 percent decaf. The difference in flavor and effect was negligible, so we thought we could beat this drug—no problem. The second week we cut our caffeine intake to 50 percent. We had slight headaches, but thought we were not getting enough sleep. We were not yet ready to admit the true cause. We continued our regimen cutting the amount of caffeine to 25 percent on the third week. It was harder to wake up every morning, and my eyelids felt heavy all day. Mary began complaining that her muscles and head ached. She felt tired and irritable. We argued over things that were incredibly trivial. I got angry for no reason. I was edgy, depressed, and felt like hell. The plan that had seemed so simple had become a challenge. Mary and I, both lawyers, could not focus at work and were becoming much less productive. Thoughts of coffee were constantly occupying our minds.

One day Mary had overlooked a crucial aspect of the case and neglected to request an essential document. Had the brief been submitted without it, the client's chances of winning would have been seriously harmed.

That evening Mary came home in a rage. She was shaking as she yelled, "I curse the day when I agreed with your idiotic idea. I can't focus. I can't function. I need caffeine!" She popped her eyes out furiously. "I can't do it any longer."

I felt bad seeing her so upset. I agreed. I, too, barely could continue. What seemed like an innocent challenge at first, turned out to be a terrible ordeal. After close to three weeks of efforts, we decided to give up on giving up coffee. Neither of us wanted to admit failure, but we had failed. We tried to quit again in the summer when we had a break from work, but it turned out to be just as difficult. Perhaps we were not ready to quit.

The problem with caffeine is that once you are addicted, you feel like you have lost control if you don't drink it, but you also feel like you have lost control because you cannot stop drinking it. I wish someone had warned me that caffeine is an addictive drug when I started to drink coffee in law school. Instead, I just heard students joke around about how much coffee they drank, how much they "love the mug," and how it would help them to survive law school. I cannot change the past; I can only improve the future. I felt I had to do something to get my freedom back, but at the same time, I felt an inability to do anything. I couldn't quit, at least for now.

The next morning I woke up at seven a.m. sharp to grind a fresh batch of coffee beans. How quickly the aroma permeated our apartment! Mary shouted from the bedroom in a hopeful voice, "Coffee? Is that real coffee?"

"Yes, come and get it!" I replied. We had given in.

There we stood, in front of Mr. Pot, two lost addicts, anxiously looking at the falling drops, recognizing our problem as we continued to deny it. We grabbed hold of our mugs, shared a guilty, knowing glance, and poured two full mugs of 100 percent pure coffee. Burning our tongues, we took a sip. "Ahh, that's good!" Mary said. Yes, it was good. More than good. It was great. It created a rush. Just then, it became clearer than ever how potent this drug is and how painful withdrawal can be. It was also on this morning when I realized how addicted we both were. Neither of us could deny it nor laugh it off anymore. We were truly caffeine addicts. If a single cup of coffee can make you feel that good, there is something seriously wrong. Having to rely on a substance to function properly during the day means something is seriously wrong. I blame myself for having treated the problem so flippantly all these years. I realized that it would take more effort, discipline, and commitment to quit than I ever thought. It's worth trying.

~ 24th Confession ~
Reincarnation

I started "doing" caffeine at age 12. I say "doing" caffeine because of how much I abused it, or better yet, how much it abused me. I started by drinking coffee. Not that I liked it. I drank it for the effect it had on me.

Coffee was an addiction. I could not spend a day without coffee. I needed caffeine because I was constantly tired. No matter how long I slept at night, I woke up tired the next morning. I would down two to four cups of coffee to revive myself, but after 15 minutes of being awake, I would drop back into a tired oblivion, dragging everywhere I went.

I had a condition called Gastro Esophageal Reflux Disease (GERD), in which the esophagus does not close completely. I was not aware that coffee caused my gastric system to go haywire, so I never thought to quit for that reason.

I didn't admit I had a caffeine addiction until my wife said I couldn't quit. To prove her wrong, I tried. The first day, I felt tired and had a slight headache, but I took naps and congratulated myself on how easy it was. The second day, I woke up with a head-splitting migraine. I was in a foul mood all day and snapped at anyone who crossed my path. I decided quitting was not for me and accepted my wife's "I told you so" instead of putting up with the pain.

When my wife, a medical student, brought home reports on caffeine's effects on one's body and mind, I decided to try again. The experience was just as bad as the first time. I was in pain, depressed, and made my family miserable. I failed again.

Then one memorable day, I was riding my scooter to work. I tried to avoid a car that had pulled out in front of me and lost my balance. I shattered my wrist, broke my ribs and a toe, hit my head on the pavement, and had severe abrasions on my body. I was delivered to the emergency room in a semiconscious state.

I remember very little of the following three months. I was under potent painkillers until treatment was over. When my head started to clear, I realized I was at peace for the first time in 28 years. I was finally caffeine-free.

The tranquility is incredible. I feel calm instead of wired, nervous, and edgy. My perception of the world is entirely different. I am a new man.

~ 25th Confession ~
Summer in the Village

I was looking forward to moving to Vancouver where I had been accepted into journalism program. I planned to live near the college, but for the summer I stayed with my parents, comforted by the thought that it was only short-term.

I found a job at a landscaping company. Every morning I would wake up at 5:30 a.m., fill my large thermos with coffee, and drive to work. At the shop, we would load the lawnmowers on the truck, stack gardening tools and our lunches in the backseat, and drive to the first stop of the day. Most of the clients were retirement residences, with their small patches of grass in the back and front yard. It would take for our team an entire day to cut the grass in the whole complex; there were hundreds of units. The work was hard: pushing a mower back and forth all day, yanking weeds, walking miles for eight or nine hours. I was exhausted, falling into bed after supper.

Then I met my first boyfriend. I had never dated much; I could barely muster up the courage to look a guy I liked in the eye. I was attractive, smart, and funny, but intensely shy and anxious in social situations. I ran into Bryan at a party. We chatted all evening and he left with my phone number.

To my surprise, he called me. Soon we were seeing one another five or six times a week. It was wonderful, but I worked nine hours a day at a physically demanding job that left me drained at the end of the evening. How could I spend almost every night until the sun came up with Bryan? My solution was caffeine pills—Wake Ups, small white packets with a rooster on the front. They were almost comical, and surely not anything to worry about. If I could buy them over-the-counter, how dangerous could they be? Thanks to Wake Ups, I could stay out all night, come home near dawn, grab an hour of sleep, and get up and head to work. My body ached, my feet were heavy, and I dreaded getting out of bed, but I was in love. That first, delirious, do-anything-to-see-you type of love.

I took Wake Ups all day, every day. After work I would eat a hurried dinner and pop two more. After a month, two did not do much, so it was four, and finally five, so that I could be wide awake to see a movie with Bryan or sit on the beach until dawn.

Then odd things started to happen. I would tell a story that I had already told. I forgot appointments, plans with friends, and was constantly rushing to an engagement late because it had slipped my mind. I would wake up in the middle of the night in a panic because I slept through plans with Bryan. My mom told me that when he called, she shook me, trying to awaken me, but I was out cold. I would snap at her for not waking me, then feel guilty. I became withdrawn and irritable. I never told my parents about the Wake Ups because I knew they would worry.

I lost ten pounds, which on my already tiny frame made me look gaunt. I was not eating well and had no energy. The initial bursts I got when I started taking the pills were long gone. By the end of the summer, my nerves were ragged, I was getting heart palpitations, Bryan and I were fighting, and I'd had enough of Wake Ups.

At first I just gave up the caffeine pills. I still had coffee in the morning, but it made me feel anxious and distracted, just like the pills. I switched to chamomile tea, so I would have something hot to sip.

Without caffeine, I was tired and grumpy. Many times I almost buckled and had coffee before work, dreading the prospect of a day of pushing a lawnmower with no caffeine. Then I remembered the racing heart, the anxiety, and guilt. I stocked up on non-caffeinated teas and stuck it out.

I started reading about the effects of coffee. I already knew it could cause anxiety, but not that it could elevate stress. If I felt stressed, my stomach would cramp. Exams or large social gatherings would have me sitting in the restroom for a good half hour. I suffered from a nervous stomach for the past few years. I popped anti-acids regularly and stayed away from what I thought was the root of my problem: spicy foods. Now I realize it was probably coffee. I have not had any stomach or bowel problems since I quit coffee.

After my summer of landscaping, I returned to school. Right away, I thought about coffee. Would I be able to study without it? Drinking coffee was a social event as well. We'd meet in groups at coffee shops to talk or study. I chose herbal tea instead. I found that as long as I had herbal tea, I could sit at the coffee shop or through any lecture.

I was a lucky caffeine junkie because I hated the effects the caffeine pills had on me and I never liked the taste of coffee. When I quit, I missed the alertness it gave me, but never the taste. I was like an alcoholic who drinks to get drunk.

Four years ago, I got married. Not to Bryan, though we remained friends. I can only vaguely recall the fun times, our dates together, and what we talked about on the beach. I still feel bad that I gave up so many memories of my first love just to stay awake.

~ 26th Confession ~
Graduating from Caffeine

My relationship with caffeine began when I was in college. I had just left the Air Force and was returning to school to complete a degree. I did not have a scholarship or piles of money just sitting around, so I had to pay my own way. I took out student loans and got a job.

I supervised a graveyard shift six days a week from 11:30 p.m. to 8
a.m. As soon as I punched out, I drove back to town and attended class until two or three in the afternoon. By the time I went to bed, I had been awake a minimum of 17 hours.

I did not have the stamina to stay awake through class. My notes looked like something a person adrift in a lifeboat would write as exposure to the elements finally took its toll.

I recall sitting through a class as fatigue set in. I heard the professor say, "The first person to bring me one of Mr. Long's ears when his head hits the table gets an A." That woke me up just as quickly as a double-shot of espresso. When I explained my situation, the professor said, "I had the same problem when I went to college, so feel free to take a nap in my class. You'll get no grief from me." Not catching grief was one thing, but not having a full understanding of the subject matter was another.

The easiest way to combat fatigue seemed to be caffeine. I had never been much of a coffee drinker, so when I started

139

drinking it, the effect was noticeable. But soon a cup of coffee was not enough, so I bought an insulated mug that held 32 ounces. When that did not suffice, I added caffeine pills. Every morning I would pour myself a gigantic cup of coffee. Then I would pop two NoDoz pills. If I had a long break between classes, I would swing by the university center for a coffee refill. I always kept caffeine pills in my backpack for the days when the usual dose wasn't enough. For a while it worked. The worst side effect was occasional shakes. When I had so much caffeine that I could not sleep, I would try to cancel the coffee's effects with a couple of beers.

It was a five-year ordeal—coffee, caffeine pills, and classes. Just for the sake of avoiding burnout, I would skip the summer semesters and try to keep my caffeine intake to a minimum. By the time my final semester began, my mother, worried about the long-term effects of my daily routine, decided to dip into her savings and pay for my tuition.

But I found it hard to give up caffeine. Putting away the pills was not a problem, but coffee was another story. I did not think of it as an addiction, just an acquired taste. My first thought was to switch to decaf; that was when the headaches started. I had heard people talk about "caffeine headaches," but I always considered these headaches to be a myth—something concocted by people who wanted to seem more important than they were and liked to brag about their coffee-fueled hectic lifestyle.

I had sinus issues, so I assumed I was having a worse time than usual with allergies. However, when my wife, a nurse, suggested that my switch to "unleaded" coffee might be the culprit, I decided to test her theory. I soon discovered that a cup of coffee or a diet soda each day kept the headaches away.

I decided I would continue to consume caffeine but in moderation. So I made a rule: no caffeine after dinner. This seemed to be a logical way to avoid the headaches caused by caffeine "deficiency" and also avoid insomnia caused by too much caffeine. For a while, this method worked. Then came fatherhood. Our child was not a good sleeper. I soon found myself having trouble staying awake at work.

At the time, I was producing commercials for a television station. The only thing more prevalent than cameras in a TV station is coffeemakers. Most people, myself included, keep one in their own office. I would start my day with a cup at home, fill my travel mug for the drive to work, and then brew a pot when I got to my office. As long as I stuck to my "none past dinner" rule, I was usually able to sleep on the nights when it wasn't my turn to deal with my son "colic-boy," as I began calling him.

In the back of my head, I knew the amount of caffeine I consumed was not healthy. My doctor had noticed a slight elevation in my blood pressure. I had lost my father and one grandfather to heart disease. So I decided that the time had come to cut back, if not to cut out, my caffeine intake.

Instead of going cold turkey, I decided to gradually cut back on coffee and diet soda. This allowed me to reduce the amount of caffeine that I ingested while avoiding the headaches. My caffeine intake was lower, but my insomnia returned. A doctor told me that my dependence on caffeine combined with my schedule (night shifts and five years of 17- or 18-hour days) caused my sleep hormones to be out of balance. He suggested an over-the-counter supplement called melatonin. It took two or three bottles, but I eventually could sleep.

Insomnia was only part of the problem. As I got closer to 40, I noticed that I was having trouble in understanding people when they talked, unless I was looking directly at them. I also noticed ringing in my ears. When I spoke to my doctor about it, he wrote it off as a sinus problem, since at the time there was a build up of fluid in my ears. He gave me a prescription-strength decongestant and sent me on my way. I took the pills and the fluid drained, but the ringing remained.

My doctor told me that tinnitus was a side effect of prolonged use of caffeine, but it usually does not manifest itself until much later in life and only if people continue to abuse caffeine well into their 50s and 60s. However, considering the amounts of caffeine that I had been taking just to get through the day in my 20s, it was the doctor's opinion that I had accelerated the process.

"Enjoy that ringing," he said, "because you're going to be hearing it for the rest of your life."

I wish I could say I am 100 percent off caffeine. I still allow myself a small cup of coffee in the morning, but I have water with meals. I have never had an energy drink and the ridiculous prices at coffeehouses keep me away. The coffeemaker that was once in my office is now in a box somewhere in the basement.

To fight drowsiness during the day I adhere to a strict bedtime schedule and do not have a TV in the bedroom. I also keep a steady regimen of jogging and weight lifting. I have three young children, so keeping them in a routine helps me stay on mine. Furthermore, my wife encourages me because her experiences as a nurse have shown her the effects of too much caffeine.

In retrospect, it is hard to imagine how I would have graduated from college without the excessive use, or some might say the abuse, of caffeine. I see kids gulping down energy drinks and claiming they cannot get through their busy days without them. To me, it is disconcerting. They have chosen the same lifestyle I chose, but with a six-to-eight-year head start. My caffeine abuse led to insomnia and permanent hearing damage, and they are setting themselves up for the same problems if not more. I was able to step away from large doses of caffeine before other serious side effects had a chance to kick in. I hope their parents are not too wrapped up in their own caffeine-fueled lifestyles to notice the damage their children are doing to themselves.

~ 27th Confession ~
Not Even Decaf

It began innocently enough. I used to work in a large office building with a Starbucks on the ground level. I've always been somewhat daunted by their lengthy and diverse menu of drinks, many of which I didn't even know how to pronounce. So when co-workers would ask me to run downstairs with them for a coffee and some harmless gossip, I would always order a vanilla steamer. That's right: I, a grown-up, would order warm milk. It tasted good, it helped calm my sometimes over-wrought nerves, and it wasn't expensive. In my hundreds of trips to that Starbucks, I have never heard anyone else order steamed milk without coffee.

Then one day, one of my co-workers, Mario, offered me a taste of his mocha with mint. It smelled heavenly, and I really liked the guy, so I took a sip. It was delicious, rich and sweet. The pink-haired barista asked if I wanted one, and I said yes. I gratefully accepted her offer of whipped cream and, ignoring the potential for third-degree burns on my tongue, gulped the whole piping-hot drink down on the six-minute walk back up to my office. I feared Mario would think I was uncouth, but I noticed he also tossed his empty cup into the trash bin outside our office doors.

By noon I was sweating and my heart was racing. I couldn't figure out why. It didn't occur to me that my first real brush with caffeine might be the cause. I'd had my share of sodas, usually 7-Up or ginger ale, but I avoided coffee and dark soda because I didn't want to yellow my teeth. I also thought coffee was too bitter. The mint mochas from Starbucks were different and delicious. I found that most mornings I didn't even want my cereal bar after drinking a cup; it was that filling. I started losing a little weight, not realizing what I know now: Most diet pills contain caffeine as an appetite suppressant.

After a few weeks, I started craving mocha in the afternoon, too. If I didn't go downstairs to Starbucks and get one, my co-workers joked that I got cranky. I definitely needed the pick-me-up and assumed it was the chocolate syrup, the mint, the flavor, or perhaps the sugar that gave me that much-needed lift.

Then I started drinking coffee on weekends. There wasn't a Starbucks in my neighborhood, but there was a Caribou Coffee, so I started going there on Saturday mornings and sometimes in the afternoons, and on Sundays, too. I got to know the baristas and who was the most generous with the whipped cream. They would begin preparing my drink when I walked in, before I even ordered it. I thought that was cool, in a "cheers" sort of way.

I lost a few more pounds. I had trouble sleeping. If I skipped a cup of mocha for a day, I got horrible headaches and became a crabby, miserable wretch. I chalked it up to stress at work. I never thought I might be addicted to the caffeine in my new drink of choice. Everyone I knew drank coffee nonstop and never had any complaints, and certainly no one seemed like an addict.

One night I woke up from a crushing pain in my chest and could not breathe. My heart was racing. I used yoga breathing and gradually calmed down. As I tried to fall asleep again, I resolved to call my doctor in the morning and schedule an appointment. Heart problems run in my family, so I could not take any chances.

By morning I had forgotten about the pain. I stopped at Starbucks on my way into the office and ordered my usual

146

mocha with mint. I walked to the elevator with the warm white cardboard cup in my hand, blissfully unaware that the reason for my recent health problems and mood swings had just cost me nearly six dollars. By the time I reached my floor, the mocha was gone, and I was licking the last little flecks of whipped cream from the lid. I had another cup after lunch, and then I went downstairs to get one more, and then one more. When I returned to my desk, I began feeling jittery. My hands shook and I could not punch the right keys. My mind was running faster than my hands. I skipped letters and words. I felt cranky and nauseous. I was sweating and I had chest pains. I left the office early. On the way home, I stopped at Caribou for one more mocha.

At night I woke up from twitchy legs and a painful, frightening, irregular heartbeat. The next morning I did remember to call my doctor. His receptionist scheduled the appointment for the following week. I told her I had been having trouble sleeping and that when I finally did fall asleep, I would wake up from cramps in my legs and heart palpitations. I did not tell her that I was afraid that it was heart disease; I was too scared to say the words out loud. With a laugh she said, "Honey, lay off the coffee." I didn't think she was giving me advice.

When I walked into Starbucks later that morning, I paused. It occurred to me that these drinks might be causing some of my problems. I had heard growing up, like probably almost all children, that caffeine might stunt your growth and that it made some people hyper, but I didn't know anything else about it. I thought I would ask the doctor about it. In the meantime, I ordered a smaller size cup of mocha. Soon I was cravings another one, but I was too busy to run downstairs. By noon I was hit with a blinding headache. I took two Tylenol for Migraines tablets and had a cup of mocha and felt much better. I stopped at Starbucks again on the way home.

I couldn't fall asleep until almost three o'clock in the morning. Then I woke up—my heart was racing. I woke up two more nights in a row before the doctor's appointment on Monday. By the time I arrived at his office, I was terrified but resigned, certain he would tell me that I, at age 28, would need a pacemaker. Instead, he asked me about my work, my dating life, my exercise, and my diet, particularly alcohol and caffeine. I was surprised and said, "I thought your receptionist was joking."

"No," he said, with a calm smile, "she might be right." He advised me to stay away from coffee to see if that helped and warned me that I might have some unpleasant side effects from the withdrawal: headaches, moodiness, nervousness, or gain a little weight. He made it sound as though it would be a struggle when he said, "Try your best not to give in." I must have looked skeptical, because he said, "I'm serious. It may not be as easy as you think."

The next morning I held my breath as I walked by Starbucks to avoid the tempting aroma. I ate my cereal bar for the first time in months, and when Mario stopped by my office door to see if I wanted a coffee, I declined. I tried not to think about coffee the next few days. My doctor had been right; this was not going to be easy.

Three days later, Mario asked what was going on. Why was I hiding? Was I mad at him?

"Mario," I started, taking a deep breath, "I'm hooked on coffee, actually on caffeine. I'm trying to quit." It sounded crazy when I blurted it out like that.

"Is that why you don't want to go to Starbucks with me?" he asked. I nodded sheepishly.

"You know," he said, "they do make decaf mochas."

Silly me, I hadn't thought of that. When he walked away to get his mocha, I googled the caffeine content in decaf coffee.

Tempting, but it did still have caffeine in it, and I didn't want to cheat. This really was going to be tough.

At a family birthday party the next day, I told my cousin about my addiction, but she didn't bat an eye. She's a Mormon, and she told me that Mormons avoid caffeine, just like they avoid cigarettes and alcohol and everything else addictive.

"Look out," she advised. "Many over-the-counter medications also contain caffeine."

"Like what?" I asked, mystified.

"Well, like Tylenol for Migraines," she said.

Aha! That's why that stuff worked so well in getting rid of my headaches.

My cousin continued with her list of the places caffeine pops up: not just in energy bars and drinks, but in some lip balms and sunflower seeds. By then I wasn't really listening. I was still annoyed that I had been cheating with my headache medicine without even knowing it.

After three weeks, I went back to my doctor. My blood pressure was a little lower. I had gained six pounds. I told him I was feeling much better.

"Great," he said. "Now let's talk about your cholesterol..."

When he asked about my withdrawal process, I did not tell him about Tylenol.

Since I quit, I go to Starbucks and order my vanilla steamer. The pink-haired barista smiles as she makes it. She can smile as much as she wants, but mint mochas are not worth heart palpitations, restless legs, sleepless nights, and morning headaches.

In spite of my fervent avoidance of all caffeine-containing products, I haven't become a social outcast. When my now-boyfriend, Mario, offers me a sip of his own decaf mocha with mint, I sweetly request a peck on the cheek instead.

~ 28th Confession ~
The Call of Coke

"I love Coke."

Around me, headset-crowned heads turned to see who had professed such an illegal love. My supervisor stood up from his desk. "Mr. J.," he said, "step into my office."

My heart was racing, almost jumping out of my shirt. Sweat collected at my hairline and threatened to drip down my forehead. My undershirt was damp and clinging. My hands twitched. None of this was from anxiety. I was in the first hour of my shift, just back from lunch, where I had consumed a diet pill and half a dozen cans of my favorite drink.

In the office, I took a seat, rocking back and forth, my fingers still striking at phantom keys.

"Mr. J., comments like that are inappropriate."

It hit me. "Oh, no; I meant Coca-Cola. I love it." I realized too late the double entendre of what I had said. I felt my face flush, though I was not embarrassed. The diet capsule was releasing its 200 milligrams of caffeine. I felt high. Caffeine had transformed me from an inherent type B personality to a type A.

My supervisor was watching me. His face said he was not buying my explanation.

"I want you to take a drug test," he said.

"What? I have never done drugs in my life, and I am not taking a test to prove it," I raised my voice.

He held up a hand to stop my protest. "I can't force you to," he replied, "but if I think your behavior represents a threat to your coworkers, I can give you your walking papers." Keeping a wary eye on my rocking frame, he jabbed the intercom on his desk and called for security to escort me out. "You can collect your paycheck and the contents of your desk tomorrow," he said.

A moment later, I marched my walk of shame alongside my coworkers' desks. Wide-eyed, everyone was watching me and whispering to one another.

Only two months out of college and one week into my first job, I had already etched a permanent black mark on my resume.

Outside the building, I caught my reflection in the glass door. Beyond overweight, I had not dated in years because of sagging body and increased tendency to sweats. Shaking like an off-balance washing machine, all I could think of was the six-pack of Coke in my desk drawer.

For years, Coca-Cola had been the center of my life. To my mother, nutrition was very important—three square meals and no cartoons unless you ate your vegetables. To save my teeth, candy was a holiday treat, and soda of any kind was particularly rare. When I entered junior high, I was granted greater freedom. I could have one Coke a week—but just one. My mother stood firm, forbidding refills. My weeks became like a long tunnel, and all I saw was the Coke at the end. I had to find a way to get more.

I received some spending money, but it was as a parent credit line. I could not buy anything solo. I was sure to pick up any change I saw on the ground, but the coins were too few and far between. I remembered that my mother kept a change jar on her desk. For two quarters, I could have 12 ounces of the most wonderful drink I had ever tasted.

For a week I was in heaven. Then there were no more silver coins buried in the copper pile. I pondered how to get at the Coke in the vending machines at school. Without Coke, I was wracked with headaches and drowsiness. I snapped at friends and was impatient with teachers. As my outbursts got worse and my grades suffered, I knew I had to act.

The only other source of money was my mother's purse. I watched until I knew I would have enough time to take some. I took a five. I did the same thing every few days after that. I built up a nest of cash that saw me through the rest of junior high.

In high school, lunches cost five dollars a day. I told my parents they cost ten. The difference became my Coke fund. I began to really feel Coke's call. When I drank one, I would grab the edge of the table with both hands, close my eyes, and control my breathing until I could feel the caffeine take hold.

With easy and plentiful access to Coke, I soon became accustomed to my regular level of caffeine and needed to increase my dose. Every day I bought one extra can, smuggled it home, and kept it hidden.

When everyone else was asleep, I pulled it out. Alone in the dark, I fed my addiction.

I arrived at college with sheets for the dorm bed and a 12-pack of Coke. Books, my computer, and a TV all came later. Living on campus gave me the most freedom I had ever experienced. Dorm food was prepaid and all-you-can-eat, and there was a soda fountain where ice-cold Coke flowed without end. I would fill five glasses and put them all on my tray at once. I also filled bottles to take back to my room. I drank Coke every morning. I could skip breakfast, but I could not begin a day without Coke. The soda fountain drew me like a magnet. It was always on, and oh-so-cold. On my way to class, I ducked in the cafeteria and filled my water bottle with Coke. I pursued an ever-growing need for caffeine. Three times a day I drank two-liter bottles, swallowed in minutes to maximize the high from caffeine.

By the end of my first year, I had gained 40 pounds. For the rest of college, I did not know that the cause was my sugar intake, a side effect of my Coke addiction. I was also unaware that the newly formed cysts under my skin were the result of my abnormal daily sugar intake.

Shortly before graduation I was diagnosed with high blood pressure. The doctor asked about my eating habits. My Coke consumption raised an eyebrow, and when the doctor did the math, I was amazed. When the doctor asked why I was drinking so much Coke, I thought for a moment. It tasted great, but I could not remember the last time I had paused to enjoy the flavor.

I answered, "I guess I just need caffeine."

The doctor sent me home with a list of things to bring down my blood pressure, circling the first item on the list: reduce sugar intake. That day I skipped my dinner ration of Coke. I fell asleep hours earlier than usual and slept nearly 12 hours. The next day I had a splitting headache.

For several days I tried to cut back, but caffeine became all I could think about. I could not read, write papers, or even watch TV without feeling the call of Coke. As a result, I consumed an additional soda later in the evening to make up for the caffeine I had skipped during the day, and that affected my sleep. I thought that with graduation only a few months away, I should just keep drinking Coke until then.

Graduation came and went, and I set out to fight my addiction.

However, my first thought was vanity. I had to lose weight. I was tipping the scales at 265 pounds, 90 pounds more than when I began college. I turned to diet pills. Each tablet contained 200 mg of caffeine, but they promised quick and easy weight reduction. So three times a day, I swallowed a pill.

Even though I was getting even more caffeine than usual, my thoughts still turned to Coke whenever I sat down to eat. I began to sneak a few cans with each meal, until I was back to drinking a 12-pack a day.

For a month I experimented with different ideas about how to lose weight, quit drinking Coke, and lower my blood pressure. I knew caffeine was the cause of my problems, but it never seemed obvious.

Everyone I knew drank soda or coffee, and they all seemed fine.

When I lost my job, I hadn't yet dropped any weight, and I was ingesting more caffeine than ever. In that sorry state, I came home, staring at my pink slip and sucking down a Coke for comfort. As I closed my eyes waiting for the caffeine flow, I realized I was dependent on something that gave nothing in return. In a moment Coke became the enemy. I saw it for what it was. Caffeine was a chemical with a huge potential for abuse. It had taken everything of value from me. I swore I would beat it.

I dug up the sheet the doctor had sent home with me. Every problem I had developed was a side effect of my addiction. Weight gain and high blood pressure were complications of the sugar, sodium, and caffeine in Coke, so I began by eliminating Coke from my diet. Sugar was my first target. Caffeine I decided to save for last, so I began to drink coffee instead of Coke. Ten cups a day would give me the caffeine I needed, and if I drank it black there would be no sugar. The diet pills were easy to cut out because they weren't working.

I planned to add one cup of coffee to my daily intake while subtracting three cans of Coke. Each week I replaced three more cans with a cup of coffee. I became aware that Coke was my second greatest expense after rent—I had been drinking 17 cans a day. Switching back to cans from bottles was important because I was avoiding the temptation to "just finish the bottle." There were times when I slipped up and cracked opened an extra can, desiring more Coke than was allotted. Instead of punishing myself for cheating, I simply extended the timeframe by an additional week before stepping down another three cans.

It took ten weeks to cut Coke entirely from my diet. I began to lose weight almost immediately. My blood pressure was still above normal, but there had been a drop.

I discovered that I was also addicted to the burn of carbonation, which I learned was a physical addiction. I began to use carbonated water as a replacement.

Once, I almost fell off the wagon. At a friend's house, we were watching football and I was offered a Coke. It was much easier to say no because I brought several bottles of carbonated water with me. All around the room friends stopped watching the game to see if I was joking.

For my next cycle, I knew cutting out one cup of coffee meant cutting ten percent of caffeine from my daily intake. I decided to substitute coffee with tea, which had less caffeine. Over ten weeks I cut my caffeine intake in half. My last phase was to switch from caffeinated to non-caffeinated tea.

I continued to lose weight. I had already lost 50 pounds and was losing nearly 10 more pounds a month. I no longer had aches and pains from being overweight. My energy level didn't rise and fall as the caffeine came and went, and I just felt happier.

I came away with a body that felt like it belonged to someone my age and a new wardrobe to go with my 70-pound weight loss. I received a clean bill of health from my doctor and had thousands of extra dollars to spend each year.

To this day, I still stoop to pick up fallen change, and I still drink carbonated water. These two things are the scars that remind me how desperate life can become and how hard it was to break my addiction. They remind me that I won.

~ 29th Confession ~
It All Started with a Headache

We ran out of coffee on a Thursday morning. Confirmed coffee-swillers, my husband and I were aghast. How were we going to make it through the morning? My husband, Fred, suffers from ADD (Attention Deficit Disorder) and self-medicates with caffeine. He claims it keeps him focused and helps to combat the debilitating effects of this condition without having to rely on prescription drugs.

Mr. Awesome poured the last half-cup that was left in the pot from the previous morning and chugged it down. "Don't worry about me, darling," I muttered, "I'll manage somehow." By afternoon I had a slight headache, which I attributed to sinus pressure. The day wore on, and I decided to take a decongestant and go to bed early.

Friday morning the headache was still there. I staggered downstairs and was searching through the cupboards for coffee when Fred came down the stairs.

"Did you make the coffee yet?" My husband sped through the kitchen looking more morning-stressed than usual.

"Did you get any?"

"No. Didn't you?"

We looked at each other, panic-stricken. After a liberal exchange of blame, we both promised to buy some on the way home. He left for work, grabbing a Diet Coke and two Mountain Dew on the way.

I had a meeting that morning and no time to buy coffee. Since I don't drink diet soda or Mountain Dew, I hoped fervently that I'd be able to score a cup of coffee at the meeting. I was out of luck, however. The only coffee there was on the breath of the woman sitting next to me. By 11 a.m. my head was pounding so hard that I couldn't think.

After the meeting I went to my friend's house rather than go home to the mountain of laundry waiting for me. Joanne was slamming her fourth Mountain Dew of the morning. I begged two acetaminophens and grabbed a cookie from the package on the counter.

Crunching away, I felt compelled to comment, "I don't know how you can drink that stuff."
"Well, I like my caffeine cold and carbonated," she stated.
"Yeah, well, I haven't had any caffeine for two days now. We've
been out of coffee, and I don't do diet soda and that's all that's left."

She noticed I was rubbing my temples. "You know, that's probably what's causing your headache. Caffeine withdrawal."

I laughed. "You can't get addicted to caffeine."

She didn't laugh. "Sure you can," Joanne said. "It's a drug you know."

"You make me sound like an addict," I said.

"Well, let's face it, we both are." "I am not an addict!"
"At least I admit it."

On my way out the door, I snagged a Coke from Joanne's fridge and drank it on the way home. Half an hour later my headache was gone. Could I really be addicted to caffeine?

The next morning was Saturday. Fred made a pot of coffee and poured himself a mug. I stopped him as he was pouring one for me.

"I'm going cold turkey."

"You're kidding, right?" he asked.

"Nope. You should quit, too. You know it's not good for you."

Fred has kidney stones. He has endured lithotripsy, and when that failed to dissolve it, he had surgery. Doctors told him to quit drinking coffee. He cut down for a while, but soon went back to drinking six or seven cups a day.

"Yeah, and pigs should fly, but they won't," he retorted. You won't either. Quit, that is."

That sealed the deal. I would show him! However, I underestimated the power caffeine had over me. By the third day, I had one nerve left, and my family was on it.

"Why are you yelling so much all of a sudden?" my daughter wanted to know.

"Why are you such a pain all of a sudden?" I countered.

My darling husband sauntered through the kitchen with a large cup of coffee. I would have killed just for a sniff, but he held it tantalizingly out of reach.

161

"So how's that "no caffeine" thing working out for you?" he smirked.

If I could focus, I would answer him. For two weeks I felt as if I was single-handedly keeping Tylenol in business, swallowing up to eight pills a day. My headache was a constant companion. I was exhausted during the day and could not sleep at night. I was jittery, groggy, and had trouble concentrating. Through the haze, I could barely make out the grin of my Prince Charming, holding a mug of coffee.

Every morning I got up longing for a hot cup of coffee. It was hard. To help the transition, I switched to tea, rationalizing that it had less caffeine than coffee. Gradually I switched from caffeinated to herbal tea.

I had never realized how much caffeinated drinks are a part of our culture. Even though I had never thought that coffee tasted as good as it smells, commercials and my surroundings made me long for the taste. So many social situations revolve around the coffeepot. I went to friends' houses and the first thing they asked was, "Do you want coffee?" Waitresses would automatically pour it into my cup. In the church on Sunday mornings, everyone stood in the kitchen pouring, creaming, stirring, and sucking down that life-giving fluid. When I announced I had given up caffeine, they looked at me like I was crazy. People who knew me best were pessimistic about my success, "You'll be back. You won't hold out for long!" I didn't understand why at the time, but people seemed to want me to fail. Somehow, my decision to give up caffeine was threatening to their own addiction they didn't want to admit.

In the middle of my ordeal, my aunt came for a visit. A champion coffee drinker, she has been known to drink three pots a day. One day I noticed her teeth were a dull tan, with darker brown lines running down. "You know, I've been wondering about your teeth," I said. "What happened to cause them to be discolored? Did you have a high fever that damaged the enamel?"

She looked puzzled before digging a compact out of her purse and examining her smile, "Oh, this? It's nothing, just years of drinking black coffee. Any more in the pot?"

As the days went on, the horrible, throbbing headaches gradually lessened to a dull pain and then departed altogether. I slept better than I had in years. I was less irritable, more patient with my children, and with Fred, the caffeine junkie.

Old habits die hard. I still craved the taste of a hot cup of coffee sliding down my throat, especially in the morning. When I sat down with the paper, I immediately found myself wanting a cup of coffee. One morning, distracted by what I was reading, I poured myself a mug. I hadn't even realized it until I took a sip. What the heck, one cup won't hurt, I thought. It did. By afternoon my stomach was roiling, my head ached, and I felt shaky. I thought I was going to be sick.

That incident only strengthened my resolve. I made a habit to walk every morning, dragging myself as far away from the hypnotic spell of the coffeepot as I could. I was determined to break my dependence on caffeine.

The crab I married was still steadfastly refusing to admit that quitting caffeine made sense. As he clutched his chest and belched one evening before reaching for the antacids, I made a disapproving noise.

"What's the matter?" he snipped. "You need one of these?" "No," I smiled sweetly, "I feel great! That chamomile tea that I drank before bed did wonders."

"Oh, you're just a paragon of virtue," he snarled.

I had struggled with ulcers and stomach pain since I was in college; now I was finally able to give up Maalox. I used to crash in afternoons, running for a cup of coffee to keep going. Now I had more energy.

There were other benefits, too. My neck and shoulders did not seem as tight. The pain caused by fibrous breasts lessened. I noticed that my mind was sharper, my writing was wittier, my checkbook balanced, and I didn't lose my car keys every other day.

Fred and I were savoring a few quiet moments one afternoon when the love of my life shifted his considerable weight and whined, "I think I've gained a few pounds."

"Mmm."

"Can you feel my pulse? My heart is racing. I think maybe I'm coming down with something."

"I think you have a bad case of caffeine overload." Putting down my book, I decided to confront him. "Since I quit caffeine, I've started exercising and dropped five pounds. We can do this together. Come on, join me."

"Come over to the dark side where there's no French roast? Never." Then, while we slept, Mother Nature, in a fit of pique, buried us under a mound of snow. The kids, overjoyed with a snow day, went back to bed. Down the stairs trundled the grumpy bear who shared my bed. He poured water into the coffeemaker, put grounds into the filter, and hit the "on" button. Nothing happened. He tried again. He unplugged and re-plugged the coffeepot. Nothing. He roared and reached for a soda. The kids had drunk it all the night before. He stood there like a druggie who needed fix. Looking out the window—as if the solution lay outside—his gaze lit on our car buried under the snow. The horrible truth sank in: There would be no caffeine for him that day.

By eight o'clock he was in bed, a quivering mass. The next morning, my darling leaned over and said in a sultry whisper, "Can I join you for your morning walk?" When we got back, we had a cup of tea together. There might be hope for him yet.

~ 30th Confession ~
Caffeine Baby

In Texas, or anywhere in the South, coffee is a way of life. We have coffee hour instead of tea or cocktail hour. My family always took it a step further. We would have morning coffee over conversation and breakfast, afternoon coffee over conversation and snacks, and evening coffee over conversation and dessert. A cup of coffee gathered us together.

Coffee was also about love and cozy moments of comfort. I remember when I was a little girl sitting in bed with my mother in our pajamas, and my dad would bring us both cups of coffee. Mine was mostly milk, but it contained coffee just the same. Every morning for 35 years he brought my mother a cup of coffee in bed. He still does to this day.

When I began high school, the social and academic pressure became very draining. I'd drink a cup—or two—of coffee in the morning before school and a whole pot to stay up late and get my homework done.

In college, my love affair with coffee grew to new heights. Not only was I working against the clock to accommodate a tremendous workload, but I was also away from home for the first time. Coffee was as comforting as a baby's blanket when I thought I wouldn't see my family for months. I'd have at least two cups in the morning before class and a cup in the afternoon, and then I needed more. Staying awake wasn't the issue; I needed to keep my homesickness away.

I discovered a place that could emotionally replace home—a cozy, nostalgic diner with a granite counter, free wireless Internet, and a bottomless coffee cup. It was the perfect spot to get away from distractions and work on papers and assignments. For hours I would sit with my computer, typing away, sometimes ordering a meal or just a slice of pie and always a steaming cup of coffee. The waitresses made sure my cup was filled to the brim. I drank seven or eight cups of coffee in a single sitting. The manager joked that I was on a liquid diet.

Never did I consider quitting coffee. It was my companion. If I was lonely, sad, or needed to think or dream, coffee was there. Some of the best moments that I'd shared with my family included coffee. I didn't want to believe that it could be affecting my health, but it was. I never had as much energy as my girlfriends. I was always tired. Whether it was morning, noon, or night, sleepiness often stood in my way. It wasn't normal, I knew, but I thought it was just me. After all, my mother was the same way.

Then I developed chronic indigestion. Almost any meal could give me horrible stomach pain, and even a simple cup of coffee could be the bullet. Taking digestive enzymes helped. However, to assume that my increase in coffee drinking had something to do with it wasn't off the mark.

I had to have at least two or three cups of strong coffee every morning—unless I wanted to get a headache. Foggy thinking, excessive tiredness, and pounding headaches were all sure annoyances if I had to skip my morning fix. I almost never let that happen.

To everyone's shock and awe, I married a non-coffee drinker. We left the South and moved to the West Coast. I was further from my family than ever before, and I had a demanding full-time job. The stress of moving across the country, entering the work force, and being a newlywed was greater than I wanted to admit. My husband, in an effort to keep going as well, began drinking coffee every morning—with an additional four shots of espresso.

In just a few months, I rushed him to the hospital with severe chest and abdominal pain. The doctors thought it was heartburn. It wasn't. They thought it was gallstones. It wasn't. After extensive blood tests, they discovered his liver enzymes were 200 percent above normal. Unless he wanted serious, permanent problems, the doctors demanded that he eat bland foods and consume no alcohol and no coffee.

Later pizza and beer returned to his diet. However, after just a few days of moderate coffee consumption—sometimes just one cup—the pain came back. When coffee was clearly singled out as the culprit, I was drinking it alone again.

I had always believed that coffee was one of life's great pleasures. I had often avoided things because of my coffee habit, such as special diets or events where I couldn't get easy access to coffee.

One weekend, our friends, who are non-coffee drinkers, invited us to go camping and hiking in Yosemite National Park. I wanted to go, but the first question that came to my mind was, what would I do about coffee? I managed to get through the four-day weekend, but I spent most of the trip feeling tired, edgy, and uncomfortable. I couldn't wait to get back home to my coffeepot.

A few days later, I got up and as usual immediately put on a coffeepot. As I went through the routine of dumping out the filter, refilling the reservoir, and waiting for it to brew, all the while feeling miserable until I could bring that first taste of coffee to my lips, I realized I was tired of the whole routine. I was tired of making coffee. I was tired of drinking coffee. I was tired of having bad breath, stomachaches, diarrhea, and headaches. I was tired of sugar and cream. I was tired of spending $40 to $50 a month on coffee. Mostly, I was tired of coffee controlling my life. Right then and there, I fully committed to ending my dependence on coffee.

I didn't tell myself that I would never have coffee again. That would make it harder to quit. The goal was not to completely remove coffee from my life, but to get to where I wouldn't need to have it.

I began gradually replacing my morning coffee with black tea. I was also addicted to sugar, so I sweetened my tea with stevia, a no-calorie natural sweetener. Gradually, I reduced two cups of black tea to one cup. Then I switched to green tea, which has even less caffeine than black. Finally, I could skip my morning tea and not feel the difference. Now I have caffeine-free herbal tea in the morning, and sometimes I don't have anything at all. I wake up feeling great instead of dragging around the house.

The transition has been surprisingly painless. I think it was because I put my full heart and soul behind it. I know that many people experience withdrawal symptoms when they try to quit coffee. My mother once tried and went into a serious depression. I, on the other hand, felt liberated. I wasn't a prisoner anymore.

To talk about ending caffeine dependence in such dramatic terms seems a little bit silly. After all, it's not cocaine, heroin, or alcohol. However, it is an addiction that affects one's health and life. It is an emotional as much as a physiological addiction. My husband urged me to stop drinking coffee because I was no fun until I had my morning cup. When I stopped drinking coffee, he was afraid that the crankier, caffeine-free me would be here to stay. Even though he was glad I'd finally quit, it was a little tense around the house. I still get snappy, but it gets better every day. Luckily for me, most of the people around me are not coffee drinkers. It helps keep temptation at bay.

While spending two weeks with my family in Texas for Christmas, the smell of coffee fills my nose almost 14 hours a day. On Christmas Day, I drink as much coffee as I want. I even have a cup or two for the few days after that, but when I return home from Texas, I step back into my caffeine-free life.

In just those few days, the effects of caffeine become magnified. I clench my jaw so hard at night that it wakes me up, and I feel groggy and tired during the day. Tea doesn't sound as appetizing, but I'm not about to throw away all the hard work I've put into my new lifestyle.

What made quitting caffeine easy was tapering off instead of going cold turkey. I substituted coffee with tea to ease the withdrawal symptoms and started getting used to life without coffee. Some mornings, the light flavor of tea just didn't cut it. I needed something richer and tastier. On those days, I would treat myself to a cup of hot chocolate instead of giving up.

I still miss coffee, but I remind myself that I choose not to drink it and look forward to that special day when I will indulge myself.

~ 31st Confession ~
Starbucks Nation

I have never smoked a cigarette, but I have been addicted to caffeine for almost 17 years. I began my relationship with caffeine in my teens when Starbucks was becoming popular, and all of a sudden, coffee was a cool drink. When I went out with my friends, I always wanted coffee. By the time I was a sophomore in high school, I was taking a thermos of Folgers with me every morning.

Weekdays were punctuated by multiple trips to Starbucks with my girlfriends. It was a silent competition: Whoever could drink the most Ventis won. Decaf was never an option. Movies and television shows that glamorized coffee drinking did not help.

A "coffee-culture" seems to dominate college campuses. Coffee is everywhere. Had I not already been addicted to caffeine when I entered college, it probably would have happened anyway. I was no longer drinking Starbucks to fit in. I needed caffeine. It had become something that my body expected; I didn't mind. I loved the feeling that my morning cup of coffee gave me. My mind was clearer, and I could concentrate for longer periods of time. The study groups I attended took place near the cafeteria, where we would take turns making coffee runs.

Soon I began to realize coffee's negative effects. Until halfway through my sophomore year, I was working out several times a week. As I began to drink more coffee, I started to work out less often. Coffee even started to replace some of my meals. If I did not have time to eat, I would have a cup of coffee instead.

Procrastination has always been a downfall of mine. I was often up all night writing or editing and I would go through two pots of coffee. However, caffeine did more than kept me awake. It also made my heartbeat faster and, at times, irregular. It was two years before I admitted to myself that caffeine might have become a problem.

Coffee and procrastination seemed to go together. I would justify putting off an assignment because I would tell myself that coffee would keep me awake to finish. I also told myself that I procrastinated, and if I did not drink coffee, I would not get my work done. My two negative habits were feeding off each other and manifesting in an unhealthy way.

I knew I needed to cut back on coffee. How hard could it be? I just would not brew any. I should have known better. You could hardly walk into a building on campus without smelling coffee. It was silly to think that I would not go out of my way to get my morning cup.

During that first day without coffee, I felt okay, but I missed the wide-awake feeling, and it was a little harder to concentrate. The next day, I had a blinding headache. I could not function. I was scatterbrained most of the morning. I thought that maybe the headache was from not having eaten. Then I thought that the head should not ache when you are hungry, and if it does, it is a sign of accumulation of toxins in the body. Since I began to detoxify my body regularly, I did not have that problem anymore. I decided to eat something anyway, just to test it out. After I ate, I still had a headache, and I desperately wanted coffee. So I made a cup. Twenty minutes later, my headache subsided. My mind was clear again. My sense of control was returning, and the rest of the day I felt much better.

I had no idea that caffeine could affect me in such a way. No one had ever warned me about this, and I had never heard of this happening to anyone. I could not believe that something that made me feel great could also make me feel terrible. However, I decided I would put off giving up coffee until I was not in school. Without caffeine, I could not concentrate and I was anxious and antsy.

Three months later, I decided to quit coffee because I started to have stomachaches every time I had a cup. The pain was so severe that I went to my doctor who affirmed that coffee could cause the pain. It was no longer fun and glamorous to drink five Venti mochas every day; it was unhealthy. So I had to find another way of getting caffeine. Soda, energy drinks, and caffeine pills replaced coffee in my diet.

My caffeine addiction was not affecting only me. My roommates had to put up with my irritability if I did not have Pepsi. My boyfriend, Ethan, was exasperated by my need for caffeine. He did not believe that caffeine was addictive; he thought I found an excuse to drink soda. Ethan wasn't a health nut, but he did not consume caffeine. I also wanted to quit. I did not want to wake up anxious in the morning and go to bed at night thinking about when and where I would get my soda the next day. I was tired of being jittery, anxious, and sleeping poorly. I wanted to be able to work out without worrying about my heart rate getting too high. I just wanted not to be dependent on caffeine. So I cut back, and eventually, I wanted to cut caffeine out of my diet completely.

One challenge I faced was the lack of support. We are a caffeine-dependent society. Caffeine is everywhere. Everyone is taking a coffee break every 15 minutes. All my girlfriends do. It is hard to quit when you are constantly being bombarded with the exact vice you are trying to eliminate.

After three and a half months, I still crave coffee, but I drink it only on a night out with my girlfriends or as a treat after dinner with Ethan, and I always order decaf. Honestly, drinking those expensive lattes and mochas makes me feel a little sick. I have found flavored teas or hot chocolate is a great alternative.

My mood has improved dramatically. I sleep better and I am a morning person now. I go to the gym and work out with no more spiking heart rate or headaches. I drink mostly water, and sometimes tea. There is a financial benefit too. Since I cut back on caffeine, I do not spend money on soda and coffee at the grocery store and on coffeehouse drinks, and I certainly do not miss shelling out six dollars for my morning latte. Ethan and I bought a juicer, so maybe I would start to crave apple-carrot-kiwi juice instead of latte.

Quitting caffeine is my decision. My friends and family encourage me, but I am the only one who can put down the coffee cup and make the decision not to pick it up again.

~ 32nd Confession ~
Ready to Wake Up

When someone says the word addiction, you might think of cigarettes, drugs, or alcohol. Caffeine addiction seldom receives the attention it deserves. However, it has the potential to destroy a person's mental and physical health. I know; I am a victim of caffeine addiction.

When I was about 13, my mother decided to start buying what I wanted to drink. I never liked water, milk, or anything else that was good for me. My choice was Pepsi. By the time I was 20, I was going through 8 cans a day. I was buying three twenty-four-packs a week—just for me. This was a financial burden, but I had to have Pepsi, or I would go insane. Pepsi gave me the psychological fix that I needed.

I suffered from headaches and insomnia. If I stayed up past 11 p.m., I was up for the night. Sometimes I would stay up for 28 hours or longer. I blamed my sleep problems on my schedule. I was a waitress at a country and western club, so I thought my internal clock was messed up. I had no idea that caffeine was the culprit.

At age 30, I started to become withdrawn. I did not want to leave the house; I was tired, irritable, and verbally abusive to everyone close to me. Every little problem drove me crazy, and I had to argue. My anger was out of control. I tried tapering off Pepsi, but it was a "must have." I needed at least three cans in the morning before I felt functional. Another problem was that sugar decayed my teeth. I had a smile of a cocaine user, but kept putting off dental work because I did not have insurance. My caffeine addiction was affecting my attention span, focus, and memory. Depression engulfed me. I was no longer myself.

I realized I needed to cut down Pepsi. I bought one pack and decided to stretch it for two weeks. I found myself opening a can of Pepsi and forgetting that I had one opened and took another one. I began to lose my freshly opened cans around the house. The attempt to cut down did not work. I knew that I had to give it up completely, but I did not have willpower.

I cried every day. I complained about one ailment or another to anyone who would listen. Something always was wrong or hurting. I went to a doctor who found nothing wrong. I started to blame everything on my mental health and went to psychiatrists, but I was not satisfied with what they told me. I knew in my heart that the problem was my caffeine addiction, but I was not ready to admit it.

One day I found out that I was expecting a baby. I felt sick. I had lower back pain and rust-colored urine. The circles under my eyes got darker. My skin was dry and pale. I had fevers off and on, and my feet got so swollen that they looked two times bigger. My hands swelled until I could not make a fist, open jars, or even grasp items. Something was wrong, but my doctor did not find anything. I felt that one of the things that made me sick was soda.

When my baby was born, I had severe headaches and shakes. I was a mess during my hospital stay. I did not sleep. I kept pacing the hall. In part, it was the excitement of having a new baby, but my restlessness was also because of caffeine withdrawal.

You would think that going home with my new baby and showing him off to friends and introducing him to his older brother would be exciting. But not for me—I was thinking about

Pepsi. I went straight to the fridge and guzzled an entire can in less than a minute. It took about three more cans before the headache and shakes subsided.

Later that year, I began to suffer from indigestion, no matter what I did or did not eat. My menstrual cycle was another problem. I would have blood in my urine three days before the start, and during the cycle my blood was so black, thick, and heavy that I considered buying adult diapers. It smelled like rotting flesh, though I was the only one who seemed to notice. Cramps and nausea troubled me regularly. Going to the doctor was out of the question. I had no insurance. Besides, I knew what caused these disorders and that my symptoms would progress if I did not stop my caffeine addiction.

My mental problems progressed. I felt anxious and was grumpy and short-tempered all day. My ability to focus was practically nonexistent. I began to just sit in front of the computer and wilt away. If someone asked me a question, they would have to repeat themselves until I heard them. I had such low self-esteem that I felt absolutely worthless. I felt paranoid. I could not leave the house. I was terrified of traffic.

The possibility of being in an accident or of something happening overwhelmed me to the point that I stayed home and locked the door. I had no friends or social life. I was living like a hermit.

I started to analyze my life and realized that caffeine had become the main focus of my existence. The way my family and I were living was not the way I wanted to live. So I quit—just like that. I knew I would have headaches that would make a root canal without anesthesia look inviting. I also knew that I had to make it through.

I figured that the first week would be the hardest, but I felt great and lost some weight. I was more patient and easier to live with and my children loved this "new me." I was full of energy, and I even went to the dentist. I realized that I had not totally quit caffeine. Because my tooth ached, I had been taking Excedrin Migraine, which contained caffeine. The next week, however, I began feeling tired. I did not feel rested even after ten hours of sleep. I felt a violent pain in my head.

I have not had any caffeine for two weeks. I still have withdrawal symptoms, but my menstrual cycle is back to normal already, no cramps or attitude, and even the blood is so much lighter. I continue to lose weight. The "not awake" feeling still doesn't go away. Other than that, I believe I am on the road to recovery.

~ 33rd Confession ~
The Last Vow

I was around eight when I tasted coffee the first time. I snuck a sip from my mother's mug. It was absolutely disgusting! I swore never to do it again. But years passed and I forgot my vow.

When I was 12, we moved to a small town in Minnesota. My new friends were into alcohol and pot, but the biggest problem was caffeine pills.

One Friday, my best friend and I decided to stay awake the entire weekend, so we hopped on our bikes and went to the gas station to buy caffeine pills. We popped two pills each and rode our bikes through the town. My legs seemed to go faster and faster. I felt free and high and I couldn't stop laughing.

Then we went to my friend's house. All evening we popped pills and drank sodas. Pumped with caffeine, we didn't sleep all night. The next morning we went to the store to buy more pills.

By Saturday night I couldn't understand what my friend was talking about. Nothing she was saying made sense. She would babble and then laugh. I laughed, too, but didn't know why. My body was shaking, my heart was racing, and I felt delirious. We stayed up Saturday night, too, but when Sunday came, we could no longer function.

I barely could get home. I lay motionless on my bed. My body seemed shut down completely. I felt sharp pain in my stomach and spent the entire day running to the toilet to vomit. I swore I would never touch caffeine pills again.

During high school and college, I avoided caffeine. After that dreadful weekend caffeine had no interest for me, and neither did alcohol nor any other drug.

Then I took a trip to Jamaica with my boyfriend. We stayed at a luxurious resort and dined in the best restaurants. At dinner my boyfriend ordered coffee. The aroma was tempting, and I was on vacation, so I tried it. The coffee was delicious. I was hooked from that first cup.

Our breakfasts stretched for hours. As we delighted in the bright sun shining down on the water and the sound of crashing waves, we indulged in coffee. The more I drank, the more I loved it. As I swam in the turquoise water and walked along the sandy beach, coffee was always on my mind.

I returned home with a few bags of coffee and the new habit. I couldn't function without coffee. Sometimes I drank so much that my hands shook, my heart raced, and I was unable to focus. It didn't stop me. I even began to drink energy shots. I liked the caffeine rush. I needed it.

I became irritable, impatient, moody, and at times aggressive or obnoxious. My mouth would curve in disgust or I would say something unpleasant. Somehow I wanted people not to like me. I felt an inner void and loneliness. I lost my inner drive. I often felt confused and couldn't make up my mind. Migraines began to spoil my life.

I used to like my job, but it began to irritate me. To overcome my inner discomfort, I found more and more pleasure in the coffee cup. Coffee helped me to deal with my surroundings, which I began to hate. I drank more coffee than anyone else in the office. I even drank the coffee syrup from the filter and ate the pulp. At lunchtime I always went to Starbucks. One day after I drank two Ventis, I started feeling dizzy, shaky, and nauseated. My heart raced and my stomach burned. I was in panic. I knew it was because of coffee. I swore I would quit, but when the feelings wore off, I ignored the effects and fell deeper into caffeine addiction.

I started buying energy shots. I was taking four shots a day. I also added them to my coffee. I like the caffeine rush.

Soon caffeine became my main focus. I felt comfortable and complete alone, especially when I had a cup in my hand. I began to lose friends. Caffeine was influencing my personality, affecting my mental and physical state, and ruining my life. One day it became obvious to me.

I was working at home that evening; I had a deadline. I brewed a full pot of coffee and was ready to work all night. I drank cup after cup and added energy shots. The more I drank, the more I felt confident I would finish my project. After about six hours, I felt absolutely crazy. I lost control over my body. I felt intense pressure on my heart. Sweat poured down on me. I began shaking. The computer screen swam in front of me. The room was swimming and I fell down. I stared at the ceiling and couldn't move.

My boyfriend came in. He shook me and yelled, "Tell me what happened!" I could only murmur, "Coffee…" He said, "One day you'll kill yourself." His words reverberated in my head: kill yourself, kill yourself, kill yourself…

Helpless, I lay on the floor and vowed I would never touch caffeine again. This time I knew I swore forever.

~ 34th Confession ~
Soda Girl

My relationship with caffeine began as a family bonding experience. During my teenage years, my family piled into my mom's white Expedition every morning, drove to our local bagel shop, and shouted our orders all at once to the poor woman in the drive-thru window. My mom always ordered a Diet Coke with lemon. It didn't take long for me to start copying her. "Large Diet Coke with lemon, please," I would shout from the backseat.

I dove right in! I began to drink a can first thing in the morning—every morning. Our fridge always had Diet Coke. When I went out to dinner with friends, I drank Diet Coke. Compared to beer and other alcoholic beverages, soda seemed to be safe. I never had a taste for alcohol, but I fitted right in with the rest of the crowed holding a drink in my hand. The difference was that my drink was Diet Coke. My reputation as the "soda girl" became established. Caffeine seemed innocent at the time. I thought I was making a healthy decision by avoiding alcohol, but I was only substituting one harm with another.

My obsession with soda continued into college. The university I attended offered only caffeine-free beverages. I didn't know how I would survive, as I was completely dependent on the campus cafeteria with its dreadful "caffeine-free Diet Coke." Fortunately, a gas station a few miles away sold soft drinks, so it became a frequent stop in my daily routine. Noting my caffeine intake, my friends began giving me Diet Coke as gifts for birthdays and holidays. But my caffeine consumption did not seem unusual to me until I was out with some friends for lunch one day.

We had driven to Utah for the weekend to visit some friends. We went to a restaurant and, as usual, I had the waiter bring a Diet Coke every few minutes. About halfway through the meal, the waiter mentioned that the other staff members were taking bets to see how much Diet Coke I would drink. They started egging me on to keep drinking. The waiter was bringing it to me by the pitcher. By the time the check was paid, I had guzzled three pitchers. I knew then that I had an issue with soda, but I had no desire to quit.

There were days every now and then when I didn't have any Diet Coke. It happened when there was none in the refrigerator, or when I was on campus all day and couldn't get to the gas station. Those days were filled with dreadful headaches, but these signs of a caffeine problem never pushed me to stop drinking Diet Coke.

I transferred to a school in Hawaii for my senior year of college and married Aaron, a surfer and fellow-student. He was well aware of my love affair with Diet Coke, but never had much concern about it.

Shortly after we were married, I began having health problems. Urinary tract infections, severe acne, and stomach pains led to frequent doctor visits. I had medications but nothing was working. I felt pain every time I ate. My face resembled the acne-ridden complexion of a 13-year-old. I put our intimate relationship on the back burner for fear that it would only reveal further health problems. I felt frustrated with my appearance and physical condition. I woke up each day without a desire to face the day and felt severely depressed.

One morning, after calling in sick to work, I found myself at the end of my rope. Sprawled on the bathroom floor in tears, I received a message: Treat your body better. I didn't understand at first. I visited the gym occasionally and only ate dessert every now and then. Isn't that all there is to being good to your body? Yet the message came again: Treat your body better.

I knew then what my body was trying to tell me: Stop with the Diet Coke. I was scared. I wished it wasn't true, but deep down I knew that my excessive caffeine intake should be stopped. From that day forward, I avoided Coke. It was in no way simple. Besides the headaches, I developed a need for afternoon naps and an earlier bedtime. This killed my social life. By eight p.m., I was done. Fortunately, I had a very patient husband. We became loyal customers of our local movie rental store, so we could stay home at night. Aaron understood when I fell asleep halfway through a movie. The headaches were gone within a week. The tiredness went away as I found other ways to stay energized, such as exercise and proper nutrition.

A few days after I quit, I was visiting my sister-in-law, Jessica. She grinned when I sat down and asked, "Want a Diet Coke?" I panicked! I found myself unable to say no when someone offered me a Coke. I had never done it before, and I literally had no idea how to start. I couldn't refuse. It happened almost daily for the first couple of weeks. Every time I visited someone, I heard the same phrase, "I'll go get your Diet Coke!" I found it striking how Diet Coke had defined me. Gradually, I found myself saying "no, thank you."

A few weeks later, I traveled to my hometown of Denver. On the drive home from the airport, my mom told me that she had the fridge stocked with Diet Coke and each can had my name on it. It's a bit sad that this was the only quality that made me stand out to others, even to my mom.

I realized that the human body is incredibly powerful. I was always persuaded that I absolutely have to have my Diet Coke, but only after a few months since I quit, soda did not sound even the slightest bit appealing. I drank water, lemonade, anything except carbonated beverages with caffeine.

My body transformed itself into the best condition it has ever been in. Within a month, I dropped ten pounds. My skin became completely clear. My urinary tract infections and stomach pains went away without any of the medications doctors had previously prescribed. I later met other caffeine addicts who suffered from urinary tract infections, and even kidney stones. When they quit, they, too, saw their problems resolved.

I wish I could say that my vow to never drink soda again was for life. I wish I could say that I didn't have a few Cokes last night when Aaron took me out for our anniversary. I wish I could say that I don't order one when I'm back home, visiting that bagel shop with my parents. After I started having a drink here and there, sure enough, those pounds crept back on. My face is not as clear as it was, and I had a urinary tract infection just last month.

I admit that I have an addiction. I wish I could drop the caffeine habit and treat my body better.

~ 35th Confession ~
Addicted to Soda

I grew up in a very poor family. My mother was addicted to soda. Rather than milk for me, she purchased soda for herself and then poured it into my baby bottle. Drinking soda in infancy and then throughout my entire childhood instead of milk deprived me of calcium. I grew up on a diet of pizza, candy, corn dogs, popcorn, and soda. My teeth rotted. At 17 I had 4 teeth pulled and replaced by a partial denture. Then my other teeth rotted away. By age 28 I had full dentures. My addiction to soda took a toll on my teeth, but this was only one of my problems.

During my 20s and 30s I averaged a 12-pack of soda a day. I also smoked cigarettes and drank alcohol. My diet was healthier than in my childhood since my wife cooked for me, but I often visited fast food restaurants.

Then one day I fell after momentarily losing my vision. A terrible throbbing in my chest convinced me that I was dying. My wife called 911. I was taken to the hospital, where tests showed that I had experienced a severe anxiety attack. I was told that if I did not change my ways, I would be dead in less than ten years.

Realizing that my health was deteriorating, I decided to quit smoking and drinking alcohol and soda. To some degree it was too late. The damage caused by a lack of calcium due to drinking soda instead of milk in infancy would be impossible to repair.

I am currently 40 years old, but I look and feel like an old man. My teeth are not my own, and I have had neck surgeries due to degenerative disc disease. My C7 disc was removed and replaced by a cadaver bone and held in place by a metal plate and four tiny screws. I suffer from osteoporosis. My bones are brittle candy, easily broken by slight impacts. My fingers hurt so much from arthritis that on some days I am barely able to type. I am a grant writer and a graduate student so I have to work in spite of the pain. I often think back to my childhood and wonder what my health would be without so much soda.

Implementing a healthy lifestyle was hard. I quit smoking and alcohol. I quit eating at fast food restaurants and began reading food labels. My wife changed her shopping habits. My in-laws changed the dishes they cooked when we visited. It was a family effort. Everyone helped. However, soda still had its hold on me. My cholesterol level continued to rise and my anxiety disorder still bothered me. I knew I had to quit soda.

When I quit smoking, I had replaced the hand-to-mouth motion of the cigarette habit with eating popcorn and this helped to reduce withdrawal symptoms. I had replaced alcohol with non-alcoholic beer. I could do something similar with soda, I thought. So I switched to carbonated water. I relapsed a few times. Caffeine is, in my opinion, just as addictive as any hard drug or alcohol. Gradually the relapses were further apart, and eventually I quit.

I no longer drink soda or alcohol, smoke, or eat unhealthy foods. Once I stopped my soda addiction, I began losing weight and lowered my cholesterol levels. I currently weigh 168 pounds, and I used to weigh 228. I run a few miles a day.

My advice is to take it slowly. Change one meal at a time. If you need a crutch like carbonated water, use one. If you need help, ask for it.

~ 36th Confession ~
Thinner Body—Thicker Wallet

My love affair with caffeine began at 17. My parents had recently divorced, and I went to live with my father. Life with my dad was fun but full of hard work. I went to school, did homework, slept from 6 to 10:30 p.m., and worked at a gas station from 11 p.m. to 7 a.m. I was very busy and very tired.

At the station, most sales came from lottery tickets, cigarettes, and energy supplements such as Yellow Hornet and Stacker. I wondered if a supplement would provide me with more energy, so I asked some customers about the supplements they were buying. One couple told me Stackers gave them so much energy they could keep going for hours. Another customer told me that when she took half a pill, she felt as if her heart would fly out of her chest. The mixed reviews did not instill confidence. Terrified that I would be the one to have a heart attack and die from energy pills, I chose a safer alternative—soda.

As a child, I never drank soda. My mother was careful about what she let us eat and drink. She had always struggled with her weight and did not want us to have the same problem. Then I moved in with my dad. He did not care what I ate. He rarely made dinner and we practically lived on Taco Bell.

Without my mother monitoring my eating habits, I went crazy. In one year I gained over 100 pounds. Not only was I exhausted from working full-time and attending school, but I also lacked the energy that natural food would have provided. Eating fast food gave me bursts of energy, but it was gone faster than it appeared, living me feeling tired, moody, and shortly after hungry again. To compensate for the lack of energy during a day and to stay awake at night, I constantly consume caffeine. Before school each morning, I drank Surge. I had cappuccino on my way home and drank Mountain Dew as I did homework. At work I would have at least six 32-ounce glasses of Mountain Dew per night, sometimes closer to ten. To say that I was consuming a lot of caffeine is an understatement; I was bouncing off the walls one minute and practically in a coma the next. My teachers were not happy about my behavior, and I do not blame them. Who would want a student who spent entire class time either talking or sleeping?

After a year of such a life, I was ready for a change. I was planning a wedding, but I had gained so much weight that I could not find a dress. There was also the money issue. I did the math to figure out how much I was spending on my addiction, and it came to well over $2,000 per year. It was hard to believe that I was drinking away the cash that I was working so hard to earn. I had no idea that I had $2,000 available to spend on something "extra" like beverages. I had even been considering getting a second job so I could pay my bills.

My best friend was also having issues with caffeine. Some days she was too keyed up to sleep; other days she was so tired that she could barely get up. She tried to limit her soda consumption and was ashamed to admit that she failed. We decided to keep each other accountable. On New Year's Day, we made a resolution to give up caffeinated soda.

The first day, I was okay. The second, I was really tired. By the third day, I was irritable, exhausted, experiencing shakes, and suffering from severe headaches. I found myself constantly saying "I am dying I want a Mountain Dew." On top of everything, I had a new job at the Wal-Mart bakery. I had to stock shelves and mop floors, but I had no energy to perform these tasks. Another duty was writing on cakes with icing, but my hands shook so much that my lettering looked like it had been written by a child. The irritability that came with constant headaches made me argue with customers and criticize co-workers. I could barely stand anyone. I soon lost my job. As I look back, I am embarrassed by the way I acted I am on the company's blacklist and can never again work at any Wal-Mart in the United States.

Giving up caffeine was even harder because my new husband was also a Mountain Dew addict. However, he supported my decision and stuck by me even when I was yelling at him for no reason. I was beginning to think that I would never get better. There were several times when I wanted to quit my resolution— my husband always had a couple of two litters of Mountain Dew in the fridge, but I restrained myself. I drank a lot of water instead. Then one day I went from feeling bad to feeling great. No wonder, I unloaded my body from foreign chemicals. Once my moodiness and attitude changed, I was able to obtain my dream job at the Department of Mental Health. By the end of the year, I was ten pounds slimmer and I had more money in my pocket. I felt like I finally had control over my life.

There are times when I want a Mountain Dew. Occasionally I even give in to the cravings. It does not taste the same and I hate the way I feel after drinking even a couple of ounces. How I used to drink gallons of soda is beyond my imagination. My obsession is gone. Mountain Dew became a regular product on the shelf of the refrigerator.

Once I got my caffeine addiction under control, I know that if I really want to do something, I can. Although it was a difficult journey from addiction to freedom, it was worth the struggle.

~ 37th Confession ~
We Get Smart Too Late

I'm a 36-year-old caffeine addict. I never thought I would be addicted to caffeine. No one ever told me that caffeine would affect me as it did or that I should watch out for it. I tried to quit many times. I am still trying.

As a child, I always loved Coke. I'd drink it any chance I got. By the time I finished high school, I was a full-blown "Coke head." I live in Pittsburgh and the colors of this town are black and gold. For me, they should have been red and white—the colors of a Coke bottle label.

In school, I devised a way to increase the amount of caffeine in Coke. I mixed 4 cups worth of ground coffee with 2 cups of water and combined it with 32 ounces of Coke; then I added a vitamin to top it off. It was my first energy drink. It tasted horrible, but it woke me up. The cup I used was a black Coca-Cola mug with gold print on it. I had that cup for many years. My mom threw it out one day. That was a bad day.

I started body building in tenth grade. By the time I got to college, I was a well-oiled machine. I ate right. I slept enough. I drank a lot of water. Protein? Check! I consumed a lot of caffeine, though.

Then I read in a bodybuilding magazine: "Caffeine will help you shed those stubborn pounds that just won't go." That meant caffeine was good for me! I was a natural bodybuilder. I didn't use steroid. I learned to burn fat with a mixture of caffeine, ephedrine, and aspirin. It was stupid, but legal and effective—too effective, and all natural bodybuilders used it. It was before the companies started coming out with "fat burners." I also used caffeine because it is a great diuretic; it pulls water out of the body. Water on contest day is bad—very bad! You could lose not because you were smaller than the next guy, but because you were a little puffier. So my caffeine intake was out of control.

Coke was still in my arsenal, but I added other drinks. The first was Blue Thunder. It was made from guarana, a plant with a high content of caffeine. I gave my brother one and he said he felt like he had just drunk rocket fuel and he had a bad reaction, almost like a drug overdose. I laughed because I drank the stuff all the time and I didn't think caffeine was a drug. I thought, what a pansy.

The two other drinks I liked were Ultimate Orange and ThermoSpeed. The first was guaranteed to make you strong. The second was a fat burner, a combination of caffeine, ephedrine, and aspirin. These drinks would get your 85-year-old grandmother out of her wheelchair and then she'd beat you with it. I told myself that half a bottle of ThermoSpeed in the morning was better than a Coke.

By this time, I was going out with the woman who would become my wife. A month before I met her, I was in a car accident. I wasn't able to work out because of a knee injury. I was getting out of shape, so I started to take a fat burner regularly. You are supposed to take it for five weeks and then go off it for five weeks. I didn't stop, so my body got used to it and I needed even more. The only problem with more is that it isn't more effective. I was gripped by caffeine.

My girlfriend saw that I was using fat burners and asked if she could try some. I gave her some Diet Fuel, a product tailored for women. Her reaction was similar to my brother's. I told myself her body wasn't conditioned. It had to be the reason; otherwise something was wrong with me. I couldn't admit it. I was 22 years old and thought I knew all I needed to know. My grandmother used to say, "We get too soon old and too late smart!" I just wasn't old enough yet to realize it.

By the time I was 25, I was a husband and a father. I was working overnight shifts, from 11 p.m. to 7 a.m., in television. During the day I had a second job at a gym. Because of work and my newborn daughter's sleep habits, I was staying up for close to 60 hours straight. What fueled my marathon? There was a new energy drink called Surge, a green beverage with a load of caffeine in it. I drank so much of the stuff that my urine was tinted green. This was more amusing to me than alarming, as it should have been. My wife started becoming concerned, but I didn't care. "Doctors stay up like this all the time and what keeps them going? So shut up and leave me alone!" I told her.

Things started happening that I couldn't explain. I had trouble focusing on daily tasks. I was starting to get the jitters. My heart rate was getting faster. One night at work, my heart started feeling really weird. It was like it had hiccups. I had a hard time catching my breath, and my pulse was out of whack. I got so scared that I started crying. I could barely move. Was I having a heart attack? Was I dying? I was only 27. Someone called my wife, who took me to the hospital. I was hooked up to an EKG for three hours, and then given a portable heart monitor to wear for a week. The doctors told me I wasn't having a heart attack; I was having palpitations. They told me stress can cause them, but they are not life threatening—just scary. Never did the doctors ask how much caffeine I consumed. Caffeine wasn't even mentioned. The stress was the real issue. So eliminate the stress, keep the Surge. I would only later find out that caffeine is a major contributor to palpitations.

The doctor suggested an antidepressant. I told him I wasn't depressed and I wasn't going to take drugs. They weren't natural, and I wasn't going to get hooked. I was worried about getting hooked on an antidepressant, but I couldn't see that I was already hooked on a different but equally debilitating drug.

I suffered from migraines. The cure was Excedrin Migraine, 130 mg of caffeine in 2 pills. I have a deviated septum from breaking my nose. I didn't know that caffeine increases sinus pain and may make migraines worse. So you are damned if you do and damned if you don't, depending on whom you talk to.

Caffeine was starting to wreak havoc on my digestive system. I suffered from irritable bowel syndrome. I gained a lot of weight from all the stuff I drank. I was worried about diabetes. I still had palpitations. I had major sweats. I noticed changes in my personality. I started to see myself in a different light. I began to realize how caffeine affected me. Finally, I admitted I was an addict.

I can't control my caffeine intake. I am weak. At first, I was defensive about being weak. My whole life I had been running away from being weak. I thought I had conquered weakness. No. I had been lying to myself.

I have battled caffeine for almost ten years and have relapsed more times than I want to admit. I can't just have one drink. I can't have any at all; otherwise it starts all again.

When I asked for support, my friends laughed at first. This had to be a joke. Then they saw how different I was without caffeine. They asked if I was okay because I was so quiet. I am a reserved person by nature. With caffeine I'm like the guy on the FedEx commercials, talking fast and never stopping. My daughter told me that she didn't like me when I had caffeine. My wife told me I was no longer the guy she had met 14 years ago. I was an irritable old man at 36. She didn't want to be married to an old man. She also figured out how much my caffeine addiction cost. I could have bought a 52-inch plasma TV with what I spent on Coke and energy drinks.

I told my wife I would quit. So I did.

In the movie New Jack City there is a scene where Chris Rock talks about getting off crack. He says, "The stuff just keeps calling me, man. It keeps calling me!" That's how I feel. I have a problem. I am addicted to caffeine. I don't want it, but I'm tempted. I still struggle. I need to quit.

~ 38th Confession ~
Out of the Woods

I grew up surrounded by addicts. My grandparents were alcoholics, my father struggled with prescription and over-the-counter drug dependence, and my mother was addicted to methamphetamines, mescaline, marijuana, antidepressants, and antipsychotic drugs. I knew the risks associated with drug use. Despite that, I turned to caffeine to get through my days.

I was the first in my family to pursue a college education, so there was a lot of pressure to do well. I would stay up all night studying. As a result, I had trouble functioning in class.

I started drinking a can of soda in the morning. I didn't care for the taste, but I loved the buzz. One twelve-pack would last an entire week. Soon, however, I began feeling sluggish in the afternoon. This was strange. Usually I felt fine. I added soda to my afternoon meal. Now I had to budget for a 24-pack of cola every week.

During the second semester my dependence on caffeine got out of hand. I was soon drinking two sodas in the morning, two in the afternoon, one in the evening, and additional sodas anywhere and everywhere. I couldn't stop.

The day that I finally realized I had a problem came five years later. I had graduated from college and moved to Colorado to pursue my career. I was drinking soda and coffee incessantly. My heart palpitated constantly. I would become irritable quickly and indiscriminately. Anybody could become a victim of my petulance. I was experiencing two or three panic attacks every month and becoming anxious about performing simple tasks. Sometimes I did not sleep two or three consecutive nights. I would try to fall asleep with no success. When I finally gave up trying and got out of the bed, I would brew a full 12-cup pot of coffee and consume the entire thing. The cycle never ended. I felt completely helpless. My life was out of control. I felt it stemmed from my dependence on caffeine, but I couldn't stop. I became a victim of my own habit.

My relationships suffered. My family and friends grew tired of dealing with my mood swings. I rarely went out because crowds triggered anxiety and panic. I had always been social. My sudden turn to solitude—or rather, isolation—was unusual.

I had not seen a doctor in years. However, it was evident that I needed help. I wasn't sleeping, my stomach was constantly in knots, my skin was in horrible condition, and I was irritable every waking hour. With much apprehension, I made an appointment. This single act changed my life.

On the day I saw my doctor, I had not slept for nearly 72 hours. She was especially troubled by my lack of sleep and my elevated blood pressure. She also noticed a twitch in my left cheek. She asked about my diet, and I casually mentioned that I consumed enough caffeine to fuel a jet airliner. She told me I had to stop. She prescribed a light sedative to help me sleep and an anti-anxiety medication that would help when I felt the need to reach for caffeine. She told me that the next two weeks would not be fun, but to keep myself alive and healthy, I had to get through it.

When I read several of the brochures she had left with me, I began calculating the amount of caffeine I consumed in an average day. It was mind-boggling. I was taking in nearly three grams of caffeine. One of the brochures explained that caffeine is lethal in excess of five grams. I didn't need to read anything else; I knew exactly what I should do.

My first day without caffeine was fairly easy. I felt a little anxious every once in a while, but I got through it. The second day, however, was awful. The sleeping aid my doctor prescribed was not working. I called in sick to work for the first time in six years. My head throbbed for much of the day, but the only pills I had contained caffeine. I tried to sleep off the headache; I couldn't. The pain was excruciating. My doctor called to see how I was coping. I explained my symptoms, and she told me there was nothing that could be done. My body needed to work itself off caffeine. She did tell me to keep water nearby. She explained that the physical act of bringing a cup of coffee or can of soda to my mouth was just as much a part of the addiction as the actual consumption of caffeine. She also told me what to expect in the next few days.

The next few days were awful. It took four days for my headache to subside, three days for my stomach to stop churning, and almost two weeks to stop reaching for the cans of soda that I formerly carried with me. After those two weeks were over, I couldn't recognize myself.

I had escaped from the cycle that was slowly killing me. However, shortly after I stopped drinking caffeine, I was hospitalized with total renal failure. There's no medical evidence that suggests that my kidneys failed as a result of caffeine addiction, but my doctor and I remain convinced that there is a connection. I recovered, and I have never felt better. I found that the effects that caffeine was having on my health far outweighed any high that I had ever experienced.

It has been nearly two years since I took my last sip of soda. Now my energy comes from exercise, and it lasts all day long. There's no quick high followed by a sudden crash. What's more, the endorphins that are released during exercising keep my spirit up as well. I'm no longer an irritable monster. My relationships with my friends and family have improved immeasurably.

I still enjoy the smell of freshly brewed coffee, but I do not consume caffeine—period. I no longer eat chocolate or take pain relievers that contain caffeine. I have completely stopped drinking coffee, tea, soda, and energy drinks. My whole life has changed tremendously. I can sleep at night, wake up every morning refreshed, and get through my entire day without feeling that I need caffeine. Now that mental space is available for more meaningful thoughts.

~ 39th Confession ~
My Elixir

Finally, I was going to quit smoking. If I logged onto my computer when I first got up in the morning, I could bypass my coffee-and-a-cigarette-on-the-porch routine. Going online seemed like a sensible way to occupy my time and mind, to distract me, and to change my pattern of behavior. I had a plan and I was ready.

I got up the next morning and mindlessly made coffee, grabbed a cigarette, sleepwalked out to the front porch, flopped down, lit the cigarette, and sipped my coffee. It wasn't until I stubbed the cigarette out that I remembered my new resolution. Already defeated, I gave myself permission to smoke the rest of the day.

The next morning I awoke and stumbled through my ritual again. Who was this person who could so easily veer from her path of self-discipline? This could not be me!

It would take me some time to identify the stumbling block. It turned out that this was not a quitting-smoking problem; it was a quitting-coffee problem. In my mind, coffee and cigarettes just seemed to go together. Once I identified the mindless behavior of fixing coffee every morning, I finally quit smoking.

Giving up coffee was more difficult than quitting cigarettes. I substituted one behavior for another by going on the Internet instead of smoking and drinking coffee, but I began to thirst for iced tea. I was substituting one caffeine source for another, though I didn't realize it yet.

I became obsessed with tea. I wanted it. I needed it. If I ran out of cigarettes late at night, I merely went to bed and ran to 7-11 the next morning. With this iced tea craze, I could not even go to bed without knowing a newly brewed pitcher would be steeping overnight. It was my reason to get up in the morning.

It took two years and pounds of sugar before I realized I was addicted to tea. I felt a bit superior over those stuck on diet soda. I knew there was no "diet" in diet soda; one could lose weight just by giving it up. Yet I could not identify my own problem. When I finally did, I stopped buying tea. I stopped buying sugar. I stopped buying little green bottles of lemon juice. I stopped keeping ice cube trays ready in the freezer. I finally got it right and switched to water.

I was pre-menopausal. All those stereotypical behaviors and physical and psychological symptoms were creeping up on me and were about to take over and run my life for the next ten years. It's not publicized anywhere, but this complex state of being, which includes mood swings, night sweats, and sleep deprivation, can be heightened and enhanced by caffeine or its withdrawal.

I began to experience horrible withdrawal symptoms: I couldn't sleep, I couldn't focus, and I couldn't think. It was easier to stop smoking. My hands trembled. My head ached. I had never really quit caffeine when I quit coffee. I had switched to tea and was consuming increasingly more cups in order to compensate for the lower levels of caffeine in tea. I wasn't even aware of what I was doing. Since a cup of tea had less caffeine than a cup of coffee, I reasoned I must be cutting down.

I wanted to find my real self, unmasked from the influence of caffeine. I yearned to sleep through the night. I was fed up with my irritability and lack of patience. Furthermore, the sugar that I consumed with the iced tea had added pounds to my body. It was clear how insidious caffeine addiction really was.

I had been diagnosed with acid reflux. The more I think about it, the more I realize that my digestive disorders were most likely caused by the acids in coffee, tea, and soda. I endured an annoying cycle of caffeine drinks, acid reflux, and prescription medicine. No one suggested that quitting caffeine might be beneficial. I had to figure this out myself.

I drank gallons of water. It flushed out the lingering effects of the caffeine. It also stilled the trembling and improved my complexion. One time my airline seatmate, a beautician, complimented my skin. "It's the gallons of water," I told her. "No soda, no coffee, no tea, just water." She knew about benefits of drinking water, but she ordered a diet soda anyway, all the while complaining about her weight. Maybe that is what everyone does: To decry the drug and consume it anyway, as if it can't affect you. Maybe people think they still have plenty of time to quit.

About a month went by before I began to find my own body rhythm, free from the influence of caffeine. I didn't force myself to wake up in the morning before I was ready. I didn't have a burning desire for a cup of tea. I didn't have the morning headaches and sluggishness. I realized that these feelings had been the symptoms of my nightly withdrawal from caffeine. Once I quit the tea-first-thing-in-the-morning habit, I found that I was just as awake as I would have been on caffeine, and I certainly didn't miss my time-consuming tea-preparation routine.

When I am socializing, everyone has coffee after the meal. "No thanks," I say. "I only drink water." If someone wants to know why, I explain that I don't want to be addicted to anything ever again.

~ 40th Confession ~
Learning the Hard Way

I spent 30 years in a state of mental havoc and physical drain. Caffeine played a major role. I analyzed, researched my problems, and came to this conclusion. The only question I have now is what paralyzed my rational thinking that I could not realize it earlier, with less blood and tears.

I started drinking black tea when I began to walk and talk. When I reached my teens, I was already a caffeine addict.

I was a very nervous child, especially in my teens. I would bite my cheeks and lips, tearing off skin until my lips bled. In high school I chewed the tips of plastic pens. If I did not have a pen, I would go back to my cheek-and-lip-biting habit. My mouth never rested, even at night: While I slept, I was grinding my teeth. I stopped chewing pens after I finished high school, but kept biting my cheeks and lips.

My hands were also constantly busy. I pulled my eyebrows out, squeezed pimples, or strongly pressed my nails into my palms to feel pain. While I was in class or on the phone, I used to draw, cover a paper with my signatures, or roll my hair on a finger.

One symptom of my nervousness was restless legs syndrome. I would twist and untwist them, shake a leg, or the leg would shake on its own as if it had a motor inside. I would walk back and forth when I was waiting for something or someone.

Sometimes in bed at night, I tossed my legs up or made crawling motions. I got rid of these nervous habits only when I got rid of caffeine, many years later.

During my first year at the university, I noticed I had difficulty processing information. I was awfully slow and felt a lack of focus and clarity. I remember a very embarrassing situation. I had a part-time job at a newspaper. Our journalist, who was abroad, called and asked me to read him his article in the latest issue—it was as if I was looking through an unfocused camera. The lines were blurry. I could barely put two words together without stumbling.

I had other awkward moments when people noticed and even joked that I was reading the same page for a long time. In one case, the person who noticed and brought it to the attention of others was my best friend; It was especially painful. I began to avoid situations where my problem would become known.

My writing became worse than my reading. I had opportunities to be published. All I had to do was to write, but I couldn't. I sat in front of a blank piece of paper for hours, drinking cup after cup of coffee, and could not give birth to even one sentence. My head was as empty as the paper in front of me. I had never realized my mental capacity was related to my consumption of caffeine, which continued to grow.

I also began to smoke cigarettes, a pack-and-a-half, sometimes two, every day. I would smoke and drink coffee, at least 15 or 20 cups per day. At the end of the day, my ears had become red and burning, my nose had turned red, and I had a weird feeling that my head had become several times larger. I smelled like an ashtray and had tobacco stains on my fingers.

I tried to quit smoking, but I began again because of my friends. They smoked in front of me, offered cigarettes to me, and begged me to stop the nonsense. This reminded me of a piece of philosophical wisdom that tells that a bucket of crawfish is never covered because no one crawfish will let another one get out. I always thought of it when I saw buckets of crawfish, crabs, and lobsters in a fish market. They were really never covered, and no one got out. So I stayed in my "bucket" for a while. Eventually I did stop smoking, but not until several years later.

I knew smoking was why I had coughing attacks that caused chest pain and mucus. The problems caused by caffeine were not so obvious. I did not know that some people cannot metabolize caffeine properly and this can cause cerebral damage, leading to dementia or reticence. I didn't know that caffeine can contribute to a chemical imbalance of serotonin. People with low serotonin levels have poor self-control and compulsive behaviors. Caffeine makes them even more compulsive. All of these explanations seem applicable to me, though in retrospect. At the time, I continued to drink cup after cup of coffee. It was never enough.

I had mental blanks. I did not know what to talk about in social situations. Sometimes I spoke as if on autopilot, unable to control my speech and thoughts. But I never thought caffeine could have a detrimental effect on my brain. I thought this is who I am.

I began to lose weight. It was so noticeable that my co-workers recommended I see a doctor. Caffeine is an excellent appetite suppressant. I was on a weight loss program without realizing it. Black coffee was my staple. I never ate much. Even when I was hungry, after a cup or two of coffee I no longer felt like eating.

Coffee was the crutch that kept me going. I felt completely drained of energy. A couple of times I fainted. I had days when I was in a cold sweats, clattering my teeth and shaking as if I were in the North Pole. I stopped going to the university and could barely hold down my job. Regardless of how much I slept, I always felt exhausted. Sometimes in the mornings my nose bled, and I was late for work. I dreamed not to work at all, ever.

Our brain is like a magnet; we attract people and situations about which we think. That's probably how Bill, my future husband, appeared in my life. He rescued me. Bill was very different from me. He was health-oriented; he did not smoke and did not drink coffee. Moreover, he did not like the smell of coffee and could not stand other people smoking around him. I knew he was right. I agreed to quit smoking, but coffee...all of my life was in the cup. I promised to try.

We got married and I moved to his city. Bill created a very comfortable life for me, not bothering me with daily chores and shopping. When I mentioned something once—simply mentioned, without expecting anything—he would remember and surprise me. He did not want me to work. And I often asked him, "Who sent you to me?"

Although I missed my friends, I thought the move was good for me. I wanted to start a new life. What I did not realize was that when you move, you take your problems, habits, and addictions with you. I did stop smoking. Regarding coffee, however, Bill and I agreed I would do it gradually. But instead of cutting it down, I began drinking even more coffee than before, probably in order to compensate for terribly missing cigarettes.

I was impossible to deal with. I could not control my thoughts and made rude remarks. At the same time, I was hypersensitive if someone said something to me or about me; I played and replayed it in my mind for days and night. Social life became unbearable. I did not want to be with people. I forced myself to be social on the phone to avoid meeting with friends. I made up stories that I was traveling. Each time I went on the next so-called trip, I felt relief knowing I would not see anyone for a while.

I read somewhere that when you have a peace of mind, health, and energy, you will immediately turn towards people. I believed one day I would. I bought a lot of designer clothes, though I never wore them. Many of them had the tags on for years. I was as obsessed with clothes as I was with coffee. Every day I opened my closet to look at my clothes or try them on. My clothes represented a world I could only dream about.

I also bought books, even though I could not read much because of my mental handicap. I could not stay focused. I would read and reread the same sentence many times over or stare at one word while mentally being someplace else. I had books I had not touched for years. I had so much I wanted to read and learn, but I did not have strength to fulfill my dreams.

I wasted an enormous amount of time drinking cup after cup of coffee, staring out the window and losing myself in the scenery of crashing waves. I did not know what to do with myself and how to break this cycle. I felt lost. I had panic attacks. The worse I felt, the more coffee I drank, as if it could solve my problems. I suffered from severe anxiety, especially in those hours when most people worked. I wanted to work, but I couldn't. I was constantly tired and barely could go through even my basic daily routine. I thought one day I would feel better and then I would have a normal life. That day never came.

I stopped seeing friends. I could not force myself to call anyone. When someone called me, I did not pick up the phone. Bill was the only person with whom I felt comfortable, except mornings. I hated when he intruded into my morning routine. Over the years, he learned that before I emptied my morning coffeepot, it would be better not to talk to me. I was not just irritable; I was a real witch. After a caffeine injection, I became nice. He could not believe that such a drastic change in behavior was possible.

I didn't know how Bill could tolerate me, but he calmly endured my nasty outbursts, not everyone could. I still vividly remembered how one morning I was in the kitchen with my stepfather, making coffee. We both felt moody and began to argue. I provoked him so much that he picked up a weapon. It was a kitchen hammer for meat, to make it softer. When the hammer almost reached my head, he slowed his hand, realizing at the last moment that he could kill me, but he struck me nonetheless. I didn't lose consciousness, but streams of blood flowed down over me. I would never forget that morning coffee.

Sometimes I felt as if I was in a semi-reality. Most likely it was because large doses of caffeine can change the state of consciousness. I did not feel I was among people when I met and spoke with them. It was like watching a play. I had to struggle mentally to get into the act.

Finally, I went to a psychiatrist. The doctor diagnosed my condition as depression and prescribed an antidepressant. I was against taking drugs. The possible side effects like liver damage or hair loss listed in a drug reference book convinced me completely. Besides, Bill knew someone who stayed on antidepressants for many years. He told me that, in his opinion, I had to get rid of coffee instead of taking another drug. I knew he was right. I had already come to this conclusion myself. I began to experience stomach pain when I drank coffee. Sometimes I also felt an acute abdominal pain on the right side. Bill told me that it might be gallstones. His co-worker's wife who drank too much coffee and took diet pills was rushed to the hospital with an acute abdominal pain and ended up on an operating table having her gallbladder removed because of gallstones. The doctors said that caffeine was a major contributor. This horror story did not touch me. We always tend to believe that something really bad happens to someone else but never to us.

However, my health began to scare me. I bought a dozen books on health and tea to use instead of coffee. The tea was irritatingly weak, and I could not feel the jolt I was looking for. Then I discovered yerba mate, a South American tea. It was strong, but I made it even stronger. I steeped as much yerba mate as I could place into a French press. I think that unconsciously I was aware that I was doing something harmful to myself because sometimes I took some tea out of the French press, added a little bit more, took just a little bit out, and then added some more, yet again. Common sense was battling with my addiction, but addiction always won.

My health continued to deteriorate. Occasional sleepless nights developed into severe insomnia. I slept every other or every third night. When I slept, it was for only four or five hours; if I woke up, I couldn't fall asleep again. It was an unbearable torture. I would have given away everything just to sleep. I seriously thought about suicide.

Sometimes I took sleeping pills, but the next day I didn't feel restful. My head ached and was foggy and my mouth was unbearably dry. I also did not want to get hooked on sleeping pills, so I took them only when I had not slept for two or three days. Sometimes the pills did not work, even when I increased the dosage. I found alcohol was much better than sleeping pills— in the beginning. After a while, half a glass of wine was not working, and I could not fall asleep without drinking half a bottle, and then a whole bottle.

The less I slept, the more I looked as if I suffered from Parkinson's disease because chronic insomnia severely affects dopamine neurons. I shuffled, my head and body were stiff and motionless, and my face never reflected emotions. Once someone called me a zombie.

During the day, I really felt like a zombie and kept drinking yerba mate. Closer to the evening, pumped with the tea, I felt slightly better, but when the night came, the insomnia repeated itself. The large amounts of liquid I was consuming, along with the caffeine's diuretic effect, kept me running to the bathroom during the night and killed my last hope of falling asleep. Caffeine's diuretic effect was only good in the morning. I could not have a bowel movement without caffeine. Constipation was my strongest argument in my battles with Bill over why I could not quit. He kept insisting. I did not want to hear it.

Another problem was that I could not sleep with Bill. I was hypersensitive to the slightest sound. I moved to another bedroom. My move killed our sexual relationship completely.

Insomnia was destroying me and my life, but I still did not connect it with my caffeine abuse. My head was always heavy. Depending on how many nights I had not slept, I even couldn't talk. I could burst out with broken phrases or open my mouth like a fish—saying nothing.

Insomnia significantly suppressed my immune system. A frequent guest was herpes, then the papilloma virus, and then demodex—a microscopic organism in the eyebrow and eyelash follicles, which causes the hairs to fall out. Although all of them never fell out at the same time, I was almost without eyebrows and eyelashes. I also suffered from eyelid twitching. I was losing bunches of hairs. Sleepless nights were leaving dark circles and big bags under my eyes. Rosacea added color to my face. I had a permanent deep red stain on my cheek. I suffered from seborrhea: The skin on my face excreted excessive amounts of oil and was covered with dry skin scales. I also suffered from acne. Dehydration caused chapped lips. Caffeine constantly dehydrated me. If I looked in the bathroom mirror right after the caffeine's diuretic effect, I was terrified how my face and neck would be instantly covered with deep elderly wrinkles, though the skin replenished itself somehow afterwards.

I was always in a cold sweat, with sweaty palms and feet, which emitted a disgusting smell if I wore synthetic socks or pantyhose. I experienced unbearably painful cramps in the calf muscles. I didn't know that the cramps and sweats were caused by dehydration, which, in turn, was caused by caffeine. I also suffered from fibrocystic breast disease and did not know that even this problem was the result of my excessive consumption of caffeine.

I became unbearable. I was filled with hate and anger. Nothing positive ever came out of my mouth. I also constantly repeated what I had already said. I drove myself, and Bill, crazy every time I left the house because I never remembered whether I closed the door and turned off the appliances, especially the iron.

One day Bill lost his patience. He called me cancer cell. I replied that before you called me flower. He yelled that he was fed up with having a wife on drugs and wanted radical changes immediately.

The next morning I came into the kitchen and my 50-pound bag of yerba mate was not there. On the table was a pile of articles with anticaffeine titles. I was furious. I threw the articles into the garbage can and began to pull everything off the kitchen shelves, trying to find something, anything, with caffeine in it. I found a few packets of coffee and boiled them in the microwave. I was ready to take the first sip when Bill ran into the kitchen and grabbed the cup out of my hands. I was roaring like a wounded animal, "Give me just one sip, just one sip." He poured the coffee out in the sink and said if he saw it again, he would throw me out of the house.

I spent two weeks in bed, hating the world, my husband, and myself. I felt I was going to die. I was in agony and I desperately needed caffeine. I attempted to go out and get some, but each time Bill stood in front of me. I stayed in bed and drank hot water, cup after cup. The first day my hands shook so strongly that I was constantly spilling the water. Little by little the shakes, pain, and anger subsided. In two weeks, to my surprise, I did not feel I needed caffeine anymore.

I began to sleep. I slept well and did not wake up at night with the need to run to the bathroom. I still had the habit to drink a lot, but I discovered that if I didn't drink in the afternoon, I could sleep through the night.

I began to recover. I looked much better, too. The red stain on my cheek disappeared and my skin wasn't excessively oily anymore. I didn't need to wipe my palm before shaking someone's hand and my feet didn't sweat so much—and didn't smell. The heaviness on my shoulders was gone.

Bill had rescued the articles about caffeine that I had thrown out and he gave them to me again. This time I read them. I was glad I did. I clearly saw that my problems stemmed from my addiction. One of the articles mentioned that coffee does have an impact on the gallbladder by inducing its contraction, and therefore causing pain. Bill was, as usual, right.

I discovered that I actually did have gallstones. No, I was not rushed to the hospital with an acute pain to discover it. I learned a natural method of getting the gallstones out. It consists of sipping a cup and a half (300 ml) of olive oil and a cup and a half of lemon juice during an evening until bedtime. This cleansing cocktail flushes the gallstones out in the morning. I do this procedure periodically, every three months, but before I'm cleansing my intestinal tract for three days. It's important.

Every three months our red blood cells renew, and the old ones turn into the green substance called bilirubin. If bilirubin is not properly filtered out by the liver, it forms into gravel-like wax-like green stones.

The process of washing them out is not pleasant, but caffeine withdrawal was not a pure pleasure either. Sometimes the cleansing process causes me a bad night's sleep, weakness, nausea, or an urge to vomit, and I struggle not to let it happen; otherwise, all my efforts will be in vain.

The next morning also may be torturous, but I'm always driven by the results; I like to see my stones, bile, cholesterol, and whatever else comes with it in the toilet. I don't want to accumulate this stuff inside me and I don't. As my blood tests show, my cholesterol level is not even on the chart, though I eat eggs every day. I also like the feeling of inner cleanliness, and I like to see that it reflects on my face. So I'm willing to torture myself again and again to attain my goals. However, this procedure is not for everyone, and I certainly do not recommend doing it without a physician's advice.

Directly, coffee or caffeine has nothing to do with the formation of stones. They form regardless whether a person drinks coffee or not.

However, substances that are toxic for the liver, like coffee, alcohol, and medications, affect its function. The healthy liver must filter bilirubin out. But who has the healthy liver nowadays when we consume so many toxic chemicals with medications, foods, and beverages? As a result, the liver does not do its function well, and gallstones accumulate in the body, causing slight to severe pain. Millions of surgeries are done every year. Caffeine, because of its stimulating effect on the body, can also be the culprit. At least one thing I can guarantee is that I will never end up on an operating table with an acute gallstone pain.

I was shocked when I read that high caffeine intake might affect breast volume in young women. My breasts stopped growing at an early stage of development. I have always blamed Mother Nature for it. I still would like to believe that it was her fault. Knowing that I might have done it to myself is devastating.

Now I loathe caffeine.

~ Conclusion ~

Did You Like Confessions of a Caffeine Addict? Before you go, we'd like to say "thank you" for purchasing our book. So a big thanks for down-loading this book and reading all the way to the end. Now we'd like ask for a *small* favor. Could you please take a minute or two and leave a review for this book on Amazon and/or Goodreads. This feedback will help us continue to write the kind of Kindle books that help you get results. And if you loved it, then please let us know. Go here http://goo.gl/P4to91 to leave a review for this book on Amazon!